Travel Well, Naturally

An Essential Guide to Staying Healthy on Personal, Business or Mission Travel

For my brother, Steve,

Be Well!

Bryan Frank

8/23/14

Bryan L. Frank, M.D.

Bryan L. Frank, M.D., P.A.

Re-Genesis Health: New Beginnings in Health & Wellness

P.O. Box 851952

Yukon, OK 73085-1952

www.TravelDoc.info

First published by Re-Genesis Health, July 2014.

ISBN 978-1500573980

Printed in the United States of America.

To order additional copies: Please visit TravelDoc.info.

Praise for Travel Well, Naturally

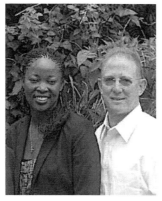

The Maisha Project has been using silver to support the health of over 645 orphans and 200 widows in Kenya for almost 5 years. Dr. Bryan Frank has traveled to Maisha Orphanage in Kenya for the past 8 years and we have used silver sol and now Structured Silver for prophylaxis to prevent, or to treat malaria, typhoid, dysentery and other infections deceases that can easily strike one on travel in a challenging environment. I personally am anemic and I take silver to help boost my immune system during my travel.

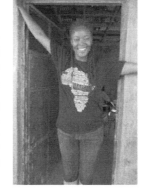

For all orphanages and international humanitarian organizations, business or vacation travelers and long or short-term missionaries, I strongly recommend reading and taking this book on travel. Silver dramatically has changed life in my community. I recovered from malaria with silver in 2012 and it can do the same for you.

Join Dr. Bryan and a Global Mission Partners project to serve with us in Kenya! You will be warmly welcomed and it may be the best travel of your life.

Beatrice Williamson, Founder, The Maisha Project, Kano Village and Nyalenda, Kenya and Oklahoma City, OK

Praise for Travel Well, Naturally, continued

Through his book, *Travel Well, Naturally,* Dr. Bryan Frank has prepared a wonderful addition to the medical armamentarium of those adventurous souls seeking to travel off the beaten path. It is well written and concise and avoids getting lost in the technical or scientific "weeds". For those wishing to delve deeper, the book is well referenced. *Travel Well, Naturally* is surely a tool that any intrepid traveler could and should pack in their travel kit.

Pamela W. Smith, M.D., MPH, MS, Director, A4M Fellowship in Metabolic, Nutritional and Functional Medicine

"Dr. Frank is an exemplary physician who is bringing missionary medical care to many parts of the world. Drawing from his many years of experience, this handbook details natural therapeutic gems that every traveler should carry and use when needed on their worldwide journeys."

Robert D. Milne, MD, Board Certified Family Practice, Integrative Medicine, Inventor of MVT-PCA pain therapy devices, Peace Corps, Paraguay 1970-73

"After logging more than 2 million miles traveling to some of the most remote places in the world, I can think of so many times I wish I had this powerful knowledge for myself and those who traveled with me. I've tossed most of my "emergency kit," replaced it with this book and a few small samples. Now I feel more prepared than ever. Bring on the next 2 million miles!"

Steve Whetstone, Senior VP International Operations for Feed The Children, 1998-2014

Praise for Travel Well, Naturally, continued

Infectious diseases are the most important consideration when travelling to many areas of the world and this book by Dr. Frank is a must have. Bryan has a vast 30-year worldwide experience with essentially all types of infections. Our Canadian registered charity, www.muvezi.org, has supplied silver to Dr. Frank and his charity, Global Mission Partners, Inc. for over five years with incredible life-giving results to thousands of the disadvantaged worldwide. I have travelled to personally assist Bryan from early morning to late evening with frequently over 200 very ill patients a day. This hands-on true humanitarian is now providing us all, through this important book, the tools to travel safely and "pass it on".

Dr. Brian Carpenter, Natural Health Consultant,
Developer of the new Structured Silver, Alberta, Canada

In today's world of voluminous information and disinformation, it is difficult to find practical helps that truly extend our health and wellbeing. This complete, concise and easy-to-understand-and-apply book will make your travel safer and your return more healthful.

I recommend that along with Dr. Bryan Frank's recommendations, you tuck this book in our luggage! Be safe, travel well and return home healthy.

Mary Schrick, ND, PhD, 3rd Opinion Radio
Health Show Host

Dr. Bryan Frank has performed an outstanding work and because of him lives have been saved. This book documents his humanitarian work and highlights the medical benefits of silver and other natural health remedies. *Travel Well, Naturally* is a must read for travelers in today's world of infectious diseases. It is truly a message of hope and love.

Gordon Pedersen, PhD, ND, Immunologist, Toxicologist,
Olympic Medalist, Best Selling Author

Being an experienced traveler, I feel this book is a must-have at all times. Dr. Bryan Frank specifically outlines methods and remedies that will aid the traveler, or anyone, with nearly any health issue. This no-nonsense, direct approach is refreshing in today's over information age. The book is laid out so the reader can get to the required information immediately. Well done, Dr. Frank; you are a credit to your profession.

David Morgan, Founder, Silver-Investor.com

I know Dr. Bryan Frank to be credible with holistic healthcare based on experience as well as evidence-based therapeutics. I commend *Travel Well, Naturally* for those traveling globally to enhance health and wellness naturally.

Adam Payne, MBA, Co-CEO Haus Bioceuticals,
General Director of Stratega Russia, Russia's largest
management consulting firm 1990-2003

Table of Contents

Introduction

Travel is so wonderful! The world offers such exciting opportunities to explore different cultures, gorgeous sites, tantalizing foods, thousands of languages and beautiful people. Whether one's purpose is personal travel and vacation, wilderness or adventure travel, business consulting and marketing or for international mission service to the poor and needy, travel abroad increases globally each year.

During my many travels abroad to trek, dive, teach or serve those with little or no access to health care, I have had the experience, personally or with those in our groups, of catching a cold, bronchitis, the flu, dysentery, malaria or some other ailment and occasionally having an accident or injury. Each of these settings calls for care out of our normal, comfortable home settings and vast resources. The challenges can be greater due to unfamiliar surroundings, limited resources or limited healthcare access.

This book is designed to share over thirty years of experience to help maintain optimal health while travelling. Even as a critically trained medical practitioner, this author's personal preferences almost always include natural approaches to maintaining health first and whenever possible. These Complementary and Alternative Medicine (CAM) therapies are often as good or even better than the common pharmaceutical approach to treating illnesses, and most often CAM therapies offer *side benefits* rather than side effects commonly seen with conventional pharmaceutical medications.

These natural approaches to health and wellness are, in fact, consistent with the World Health Organization (WHO)

Resolution 44:34, which promotes the use of "traditional, harmless, efficient and scientifically proven remedies".

A variety of CAM therapies and remedies that are typically available to most travelers are presented. These will include the new pH Structured Silver, activated charcoal, botanical/herbal, homeopathic and essential oil remedies, and various modalities such as acupuncture and auricular therapy and self-treatments for pain management while on travel. Non-medically trained travelers may often apply these therapies successfully with ease and with the information that is presented.

As this writing is designed to be easy to read for the lay public, the book is not heavily referenced, by design. A good set of references is given for those who wish to explore these further, from those references used by the author and others as well.

This book is not intended to replace sound medical advice. It is intended to present options for maintaining or regaining health and wellness on travel. *Always consult a physician or health care provider when you are in need.* What is presented herein will provide solutions for many conditions, though certainly not all. CAM therapies typically are just that, *complementary* and *alternative* therapies. As an integrative physician, I find the best care is usually provided from "the best of both worlds" of healthcare traditions.

Author Biography

Bryan L. Frank, M.D. is an integrative physician with over thirty years of experience in a US-based private practice of Anesthesiology, Natural Pain and Sports Medicine, Medical Acupuncture, Prolotherapy, Anti-aging & Regenerative Medicine, as well as in extensive travel medicine and medical missions. In his private medical practice, Dr. Frank is President of *Re-Genesis* 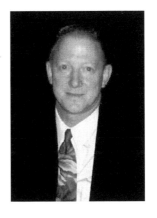 *Health: New Beginnings in Health and Wellness.*

Also as President of Global Mission Partners, Inc. (GMP), a 501-c-3 Not-for-Profit charitable corporation that serves the poor in developing parts of Asia, Africa, South America and North America, he has used the new Structured Silver, activated charcoal, botanical/herbal, homeopathic and essential oil natural therapies for maintaining health and/or treating a wide variety of medical conditions around the world. He has traveled to more than 60 countries and his teams with GMP currently serve Nepal, India, Kenya, Haiti, Ecuador and México. He has previously served in Russia, Dominican Republic, Costa Rica, Appalachia and Native American reservations.

GMP receives applications for participation in its projects from physicians, surgeons, dentists, physician assistants, nurses, optometrists, chiropractors, pharmacists, therapists and non-medical general helper volunteers, as well as students and pastors. GMP cares for those with little or no access to healthcare around the globe. Past projects, future plans and applications are available at GMP's website, www.GlobalMissionPartners.org.

Dr. Frank has extensive travel and trekking experience, treating team members while on treks in the Himalaya, below the Matterhorn, Mt. Blanc and Machu Picchu, or while in bustling cities and tiny oxcart villages of Asia, 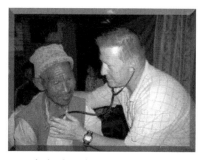 Africa and Latin America as a global missionary. He has authored the Chapter, Principles of Pain Management in the renowned and definitive text, *Wilderness Medicine, 4th and 5th Editions*, edited by the highly acclaimed Stanford Emergency Physician, Dr. Paul Auerbach.

Dr. Frank has written numerous articles on Integrative Medicine, Medical Acupuncture, Prolotherapy, Neural Therapy, and other related techniques and has written and published the highly acclaimed text, *Auricular Medicine and Auricular Therapy: A Practical Approach, Atlas of Auricular Therapy and Auricular Medicine* and reference charts for Auricular Therapy and Hand Therapy, available at www.AuricularTherapy.com.

Dr. Frank has led medical delegations to Russia, China, Korea and Japan for exchanging medical research and clinical expertise in medical acupuncture. He has lectured internationally to medical congresses, symposia and seminars to many thousands of physicians and other healthcare workers in Europe, Asia, Oceana and North and South America. He served as President of the American Academy of Medical Acupuncture/AAMA (1999-2001) and as President of the International Council of Medical

Acupuncture and Related Techniques/ICMART (2004-2006) and also as Vice-President of ICMART (2002-2004 and 2010-2012).

Dr. Frank has led hundreds of volunteers over the last 30 years to serve tens of thousands of needy children and adults in over 100 missions for healthcare, construction, street children and orphan projects, water wells, community development, women's skills development, education, micro-loan finance, as well as preaching, teaching and Christian discipleship. He has traveled to over 60 nations and taught or served on missions on 6 continents, with his teams tackling malaria, food poisoning, dysentery, cholera, hepatitis and also common ailments such as coughs, colds, flu and various pains.

Dedication

I am deeply grateful and eternally indebted to Mr. Kenshi Nabeshima, currently of Tokyo, Japan. This "Texas Samurai" led me into the wonderful world of acupuncture in 1972 while he was practicing in Dallas, Texas; he remains a faithful mentor, counselor and friend for over 40 years. His wisdom, compassion and his gifted hands have greatly blessed all who have been touched by him as practitioner, sensei, teacher and friend. The journey I began with Sensei Nabeshima began my ventures into the world of natural Complementary and Alternative Medicine, which continue to be enriched through daily discoveries to be healthy naturally.

Following this initial walk into alternative medicine I then moved into studying nutritional health and supplementation. This led me to experience food and nutrition far different from the processed junk food of teen years with the benefits of those decisions enjoyed through enhanced health and wellness. I am grateful for Texas A&M University College of Medicine Charter Class 1981 which, while it provided a remarkable conventional medical education to lead me into a pediatric and neonatology internship followed by an anesthesiology and pain medicine residency. While not supportive of nutrition and other "alternative" therapies during my training years, thankfully they were unable to quell the roots of natural healing and nutrition that began in my youth. I am grateful for the American Academy of Anti-Aging & Regenerative Medicine, through which I took my Fellowship and Board Certification, reinforcing and adding to my desire to treat patients at home or abroad with natural, non-toxic approaches to health and wellness.

Lastly, I gratefully dedicate this work to my family, patients, students and colleagues in the USA and around the globe through my clinic, teaching or medical mission practices. I am blessed by their confidence, their trust and their insights.

Bryan L. Frank, M.D.

Re-Genesis Health: New Beginnings in Health & Wellness

Global Mission Partners, Inc.

July 2014

Disclaimer

Integrative health therapies, Complementary and Alternative Medicine (CAM) and even conventional medical practices, are constantly changing through the development of researchers and practitioners worldwide. *Travel Well, Naturally* presents information felt by this author to be current and relative at the time of writing, though it is expected that additional and different insights and understandings will be appreciated in time. The information in this guide is not intended to diagnose, treat, cure or prevent disease, as these skills may only practiced by appropriate licensed healthcare providers.

Readers are advised to confirm that information regarding diagnosis, prevention, treatment, self-treatment and healthcare practitioners they are seeking is current, valid, appropriate and that it complies with the legislation and practice standards applicable to the given situation.

All patients are advised to seek the consultation of competent and informed licensed health care providers. This author and the publisher are not responsible for any adverse effects or consequences arising from the use or misuse of any of the material presented or omitted.

THE FDA HAS REVIEWED NONE OF THE STATEMENTS IN THIS BOOK. *Consult your personal healthcare provider before beginning or changing any supplemental or prescription regimen.*

Chapter 1
Preparing Before You Travel

I still always have such great excitement before I travel! After exploring over 60 nations for personal, business or missions, I still never lose the thrill of upcoming new adventures. There is, however, one certain way to insure that the travel may be disrupted, cancelled or otherwise a miserable experience; don't prepare ahead of time to stay well.

The best preparation for healthy travel will begin at least a week, better a month or more, before departure to the end of the rainbow. This should include making healthy lifestyle and dietary choices that promote health and wellness and minimize the opportunity for illness or accident.

Healthy living choices prepare for healthy travel

Contemporary American diet and lifestyle do NOT promote health and wellness, period! In fact, a common term for the usual American diet is SAD, or Standard American Diet. Much of this is due to policies and practices in the agricultural and food industries forced by special interest groups and nearly insane policies by our federal government. This has led to a drastic change in the very substance of foodstuffs over the last generation or two. Toxins and herbicides are dumped on our fields and poured into our water sources to ultimately end up on our plate. Further, genetic engineering of crops to withstand various chemicals now means that many of our crops are resistant to glyphosate. Doesn't sound ominous enough? How about Round Up®?

I shared this with a knowledgeable person who responded, "But wheat can't tolerate Round Up®, it kills plants." Well, unfortunately it can and it does, as it has been genetically modified to do so. And while gluten sensitivity is now very well-known by society, it may in fact be the glyphosate, Round Up®, that is harming people even more.

Most of the corn in America is now genetically modified. This means that as we consume corn, chips, and many other foodstuffs containing corn, the potential for the genetically modified product can and does have an impact on our own genetic expression. This is important as this gene expression can actually be directed through proper food choices to enhance wellness and resist disease. On the other hand, food-like stuff, what I call *non-food*, has the potential to lead to gene expression and metabolic damage that promote disease.

While considering gene expression, it is critical to understand that what we put in our mouths may dramatically affect the bio-flora population of our gut. The health flora of the gut, often termed probiotics, actually has more potential gene expression in our lives than our own human cells! That's right, the microorganisms that live in our gut have more genetic expression than our entire genetic code. So, it seems reasonable that promoting a healthy gut flora may promote health and wellness and diminish the potential for illness.

It is essential to take a fresh, new look at what we choose to purchase and put in our refrigerators and pantries or what we choose from the menu when we eat out.

Food, by definition, is that which we take in and are nourished. By this definition, most of what I see purchased in grocery carts in my local markets is *anti-food*. There is simply no nourishment provided and much of what we consume is filled with synthetic "nutrient" additives for the product to even qualify as food in the first place. These synthetic chemical additives cannot ever perform the essential roles of maintaining health and wellness as those live, natural enzymes and nutrients that come from real, live food.

So, a diet and lifestyle of natural, organic and wholesome proteins, fats and carbohydrates will provide us with energy, enzymes, vitamins, minerals, amino acids and anti-oxidants that support life and wellness. It is now more important than ever before in American life, to be critical and selective in what we choose to purchase. That which is canned, boxed or bagged is less likely to promote health and wellness than that which is fresh, natural and organic.

Preparing for the onslaught of bacteria, viruses, parasites and fungus

International travel necessitates that we gather in crowded waiting rooms, board crowded planes or ships and spend time with many who are either overtly sick or likely carrying disease. Fellow travelers may knowingly or innocently carry these organisms around the globe and expose us to illness. The more we maintain a healthy immune system before we travel, the better we may resist this onslaught from those around us.

So often, I have been on planes where there is constant coughing, sneezing and blowing. The airlines tell us, "it is no problem, the air is purified and safe". However, it is very likely that the germs are easily passed to many others through spread of infected micro-droplets for hours before the plane lands on yonder distant shore. If your immune system is compromised and if you have not taken precautions before travel, the likelihood of illness is increased dramatically.

Fortunately, a few simple measures can dramatically decrease the likelihood that you will be victim to this onslaught.

For starters, everyone should take a serious look at the dangerous, fraudulent and serious compromises that the US has made regarding "food". Seriously, most of what fills the grocery carts in the markets today is not meant for human consumption. It will not in any way promote health or wellness. We need to shop for organic, if possible, or do the best we can to eat fresh, live food on a daily basis. Because so much of food is literally without nutrients, we also need to supplement with a pharmaceutical-grade product. Cute colored vitamins for kids and plastic coated "vitamins" for adults will not do the job. We need reliable and proven nutrients to support our health and nutrition that we miss from our diet.

The result of a diet of natural, organic, live food products is a life of less illness, less immune compromise and less aches and pains. Eating these is a choice and we should make the choice to consume actual food which leads to health over "anti-food" which leads to disease. An occasional "treat" may be tolerated, yet far too many Americans have settled on a lifestyle of treats without any true food consumption at all. Best of all, this is the best medicine and the cheapest way to be well and stay healthy!

Next, after establishing a sound approach to solid nutrition, there are a number of remedies that can help us to resist infections, recover more quickly and generally better withstand the natural biological stresses of travel. In the following chapters, you will find the new Structured Silver, activated charcoal, botanical/herbal, homeopathic and essential oil remedies that require no physician prescription and can usually be taken in one's carry-on bag, or in the checked bag for extended travel and for liquids greater than 100 ml volume. Further, considerations for managing pain while travelling are presented, that go far beyond just popping a couple of anti-inflammatory pain medications, cough and cold remedies, etc.

Importantly, you *can* Travel Well, Naturally!

Chapter 2
The New Structured Silver for Travel

Structured Silver leads the travel remedies for a very important reason. If there is only one remedy to take on travel, it should be the new Structured Silver! Silver and various silver solutions have been used since antiquity to promote or restore health. Mentioned in the classic writings of Egyptian health practices over 5500 years ago, used by Greeks, Romans, Phoenicians and Macedonians 2500 years ago with silver vessels for water purification, by Europeans in order to blunt the effects of the plague through the use of silverware, to the last two centuries in American medical history using silver sutures, stents and catheters to decrease infection rates. Some traditional cultures (especially in India) have used silver foil as a dietary product for supporting gut health, yet some of the foil is of poor quality and it is not uncommon to see those with argyria or darkening of the skin in a blue-gray coloration in those using the inferior silver products. This is not a concern with the highest quality of silver, the new Structured Silver.

Silver kills some 650 different disease organisms! Silver products are now widely used in health care and industry with numerous applications to promote health and wellness. Space stations have used silver-based systems for water purification, as do several commercial airlines. Hospital and hotel environmental systems use silver-based systems to control infections, such as the infamous Legionnaires' disease. Silver has been used topically for decades in hospitals and clinics for burn victims, diabetic wounds and decubitus ulcers, and is also incorporated into the fabrication of stents that are used in the heart and blood vessels and in the urinary tract and kidneys to decrease infection. Silver is being integrated on various clothing items to decrease body odor or contamination in shirt armpit and socks.

Silver has been shown to interrupt microbes' cell wall function, cellular reproduction, bio-film integrity and other anti-biocide effects.

Additional uses of silver include disinfecting fruits and vegetables and preserving cosmetics, toiletries and similar hygiene products. More US patents have been applied for silver than all other metals combined in recent years, both for health care and for industrial applications. Silver is blended with plastics for lasting anti-bacterial protection and in prescription eyeglasses. Silver ions have been demonstrated to promote bone growth in fractures.

Silver-based antimicrobial biocides are used as wood preservatives and to inhibit bacterial growth in chicken farms and oyster harvesting.

Colloidal silver solutions are widely known by many who shop at health food stores, and this was a significant improvement over previous ionic solutions and salts of silver from previous generations. In the last decade or so, silver aquasols presented even further advancement with smaller silver particles in suspension, leading to greater penetration on a cellular level.

These aquasols of the last decade, and now the even more effective alkalinized new Structured Silver, have demonstrated remarkable therapeutics in both basic and clinical research for many diverse clinical situations. As this is currently the most advanced silver solution available, further discussion will only refer to the new Structured Silver. The new Structured Silver begins with structured (or activated) water, making it more energetically viable. Conventional waters have *macro*-clustered particles; structuring the water leads to *micro*-clustering, a more highly energetic solution that is more readily available for cellular uptake. Alkalinizing of the Structured Silver further offers better assimilation. Because most commercial silver solutions are not prepared in this way, they are typically slightly to very acidic.

Giving additional credence to the uniqueness of the new Structured Silver, the products have received Canada's Homeopathic Medicine Number (DIN-HM): #80046255 and #80046265 for the liquid and gel, respectively.

Structured Silver demonstrates anti-bacterial, anti-viral, anti-parasitic and anti-fungal effects for virtually every surface and tissue on or in the body. Structured Silver has demonstrated to be highly effective clinically and is without toxicity, even for at least a dozen drug-resistant bacteria. Silver solutions possess multiple modes of action. They interact with multiple molecular processes within microorganisms that result in various effects, including inhibition of growth and loss of infectivity to cell death. Metallic silver ions give off ultraviolet energy in a specific wavelength, the same wavelength that is used in hospital and food industry to eliminate microbial counts. As it interferes with the organisms' energy sources, bacteria are killed and replication in viruses is prevented. Cell wall synthesis is prevented in fungi. Interestingly, due to the lipid layer of the cell membranes of healthy probiotic bacteria, silver does not interfere with probiotic benefits in the human gut while it demonstrates profound ability, often life-saving, to kill pathogenic (harmful) organisms which have no lipid layer in the cell membrane. Even when large amounts of Structured Silver are taken orally, healthy bacteria, probiotic, populations are still maintained. These properties make Structured Silver an ideal therapeutic for travel settings.

Silver solutions have demonstrated the ability to destroy microbes, including bacteria, viruses, fungus and parasites. Studies have shown clearing of microbes at 10 ppm (parts per million) solution or less within 6-10 minutes or less, and even as low as 2-5 ppm for many organisms. A partial listing of the numerous bacteria, viruses, fungi and parasites with susceptibility in lab (in-vitro) or in clinic (in-vivo) are included in Tables 2.1 through 2.5.

Structured Silver for travel

One role of Structured Silver that may be neglected as travelers or teams prepare for business, pleasure and mission projects is that of preventing disease and maintaining good health in the participants prior to, throughout and following the travel or mission project. This author typically begins taking 1-2 tablespoons of Structured Silver twice daily in the week prior to the project, continues throughout and then following the project for at least one to two weeks. This is important, as some organisms may be latent and not expressing clinical illness for some days after return from travel.

Clearly, Structured Silver has great applications for treating travelers or patients of mission health camps while on travel as well. As an experienced travel and missionary physician with Global Mission Partners Inc. (GMP), this author has experience using Structured Silver on malaria, upper and lower respiratory infections, eye and ear infections, skin lesions and trauma and more. The widely effective use of Structured Silver for numerous infections

Table 2.1 Silver susceptibility has been demonstrated on bacteria, including:

Acinetobacter baumani
Bacillus cereus spores
Bacillus subtilis
Citrobacter freundii
Enterobacter aerogenes
Enterobacter cloacae
Enterococcus hirae
Escherichia coli
Helicobacter pylori
Klebsiella pneumoniae
Klebsiella oxytoca
Mycobacteria (various species)
Neisseria gonorrhoeae
Providencia stuartii
Pseudomonas aeruginosa
Pseudomonas. stutzeri
Pseudomonas putida
Proteus mirabilis
Salmonella Arizona
Salmonella typhi
Shigella boydii
Shigella flexineri
Staphylococcus aureus
Staphylococcus epidermidis
Streptococcus pyogenes
Streptococcus pneumoniae
Streptococcus faecalis
Streptococcus mutans
Streptococcus gordonii
Streptococcus pyogenes
Thiobacillus ferro-oxidans
Thiobacillus thio-oxidans

Table 2.2 Silver susceptibility has been demonstrated on drug-resistant bacteria, including:

Amikacin-Resistant Providencia stuartii
Ampicillin-Resistant Escherichia coli
Erythromycin-Resistant Staphylococcus pyogenes
Methicillin-Resistant Staphylococcus aureus (MRSA)
Multidrug-Resistant Pseudomonas aeruginosa
Multi-Resistant Salmonella typhi

Table 2.3 Silver susceptibility has been demonstrated on fungi, including:

Aspergillus niger
Candida albicans I
Candida albicans II
Candida glabrata
Candida krusei
Candida parapsilosis
Candida pseudotropicalis
Candida tropicalis
Torulopsis glabrata
Trichophyton mentagrophytes

Table 2.4 Silver susceptibility has been demonstrated on viruses, including:

Acute Respiratory Distress Syndrome (Coronavirus)
Haemophilus influenza
Hepatitis B
Herpes Simplex I
HIV- Human Immunodeficiency Virus
Influenza Virus A, B, C, H1N1, H5N1 (Bird Flu) and
        various species
Monkey Pox Virus

Table 2.4 Silver susceptibility has been demonstrated on viruses, including (continued):

Respiratory Syncytial Virus
Smallpox
Tacaribe Virus

Table 2.5 Silver susceptibility has been demonstrated on parasites, including:

Brugia malayi
Entamoeba histolytica
Trichonomas vaginalis
Malaria falciparum
Malaria vivax
Meriones unguiculatus

from bacteria, viruses, fungi and parasites is seen to be effective on any body surface and in any tissue. This author has used Structured Silver orally, topically as liquid or gel on skin, vagina or rectum, inhaled or sprayed into the nose or mouth and dropped in the eyes and ears. Structured Silver is well received universally and is without taste and without pain or irritation on any bodily surface or tissue.

It is not uncommon, especially during adventure travel or in small health camps in primitive, oxcart villages, to be without sophisticated bio-diagnostic tools and instruments. As such, at times a definitive diagnosis is difficult, and a clinical diagnosis or differential set of diagnoses only is available. As Structured Silver has a broad spectrum of clinical efficacy, we feel confident in using it when the lack of diagnostic resources prohibits definitive diagnosis.

Relative cost effectiveness of Structured Silver compared to conventional pharmaceuticals is a further advantage or benefit. Discounts for quantity purchases from the Internet or through qualified professionals also further good stewardship of funds through the use of Structured Silver (see Resources). GMP continues to serve and use Structured Silver to humanitarian service projects around the globe and this author also uses it regularly for business or personal travel as well.

Prior studies also show Structured Silver to be effective and safe when used in conjunction with other pharmaceuticals. In fact, studies have shown silver to potentiate the antimicrobial effects of numerous antibiotics and thus there is no contraindication to using silver with antibiotics, if indicated. With the absence of toxicity or allergy, no side effects are to be expected. This is remarkable, especially when considering the wide range of side effects often experienced with pharmaceuticals, some of which are mild, while others are quite serious or even lethal.

Structured Silver has also changed GMP's practice of vaccination usage among staff and team members. In the past, anti-malarial medications or vaccines for yellow fever, typhoid, hepatitis and others were typically used. As we now *always* travel with Structured Silver, we personally choose to not take the other vaccines and medications as preventatives. Structured Silver may even emerge as solutions for serious infections such as the recent Ebola virus and Easter Equine Encephalitis outbreaks, among others.

Consultation with your healthcare provider is essential. Further, it is imperative to take all reasonable precautions to prevent contracting infectious diseases, including but not limited to thorough hand washing, covering of nose and mouth with coughs and sneezing (yours or others), thorough washing of utensils and dishes, use of mosquito netting where indicated, use of mosquito repellents (natural, non- toxic), et cetera.

Ebola concerns

Recently, the Ebola outbreak has led to much concern and distress for a virus that ranges from 40-90% mortality rate. Ebola victims die from hemorrhagic complications and organ failure in approximately 90% of the recent outbreak patients. Even physicians and healthcare providers have contracted Ebola and are recently under care and study at Emory University hospitals in the USA.

While there are no studies on the effects of Ebola and its sensitivity to silver as an anti-viral agent, silver has demonstrated effectiveness against a wide range of viruses in research and clinic. Given the safety of Structured Silver, there is no question that GMP teams will continue to use Structured Silver on a preventative basis as we continue to serve those areas, even where Ebola is endemic. ALL travelers are encouraged to use Structured Silver to help protect themselves when traveling into areas with Ebola outbreaks. While there is no guarantee and no formal studies at this time, this should be a sober consideration.

A challenge to international travelers

Given the volumes of science, the many years of safe experience with Structured Silver, the governmental recognitions, the broad spectrum of indications for its use and the reasonable cost value, this author strongly encourages international travelers, whether for business, pleasure or for mission agencies and humanitarian projects, to seriously consider using Structured Silver on a regular basis. This recommendation includes the use of Structured Silver in field settings of village health camps for patients and also for staff and personnel on business travel or in the international health projects with regular, daily use of Structured Silver for preventive measures. The daily small use may be increased from 1-2 teaspoons twice daily to 1-2 tablespoons twice daily or more, as indicated. In addition, use of Structured Silver gel, drops or sprays may be indicated, depending on site and clinical presentation of the infection.

Structured Silver is not only useful in mission projects that are overtly medical in nature. Any international project should seriously consider the benefits of regular, daily Structured Silver use as a preventative health practice as well as prompt increase if and when indicated health problems arise. Simply stated, Structured Silver is safe, effective and cost-conscious. Management and executives of all companies sending their personal or other stakeholders in areas known to have infectious disease should make this Structured Silver available.

Stories From the Mission Field

Kenya

In a tiny village in the bush, near Kisumu, on the shores of Lake Victoria, GMP teams have served thousands in health camps, as well as partnering with local projects that develop water wells, latrines, meals for orphans and widows with AIDS, education and school support and Christian ministry. During the last five years, numerous children and adults in the village presented to healthcare providers with symptoms consistent with malaria. Malaria is endemic to the region and while diagnosis of the plasmodium in the blood and medications are available, many go without diagnosis and treatment due to extreme poverty. In this setting, GMP takes silver, donated by

Muvezi Health Projects Society of Canada, to treat these patients. Diagnosis is made and patients are then treated with 1 tablespoon (15 ml) of silver twice daily. Patients are encouraged to hold the liquid in their mouth and to swish it about for a minute prior to swallowing for absorption to begin across the mucous membranes rapidly.

In our initial trial of approximately 30 patients over the week, all patients became clinically well and were able to return to school or work within 24-48 hours, even back on the soccer field! This was often the case even in those patients that appeared clinically worse than others. Repeat blood studies are obtained and found to be reverted to normal in 2-5 days for most, and 10 days for others. Due to extreme poverty, donations are necessary to provide for the testing as the people live very pragmatically and when they are once well, they are unable to consider the cost of the test in light of needing their next meal, perhaps the only one for the day or for several days. Further testing and treatment is ongoing and it is hoped that a clinical pilot study may be published from these results in Kenya. A randomized, multi-center clinical trial of the success in malaria treatment in Africa is published in The Indian Practitioner, September 2010 (see References). While this research used the previous generation silver, the new Structured Silver is expected to produce even better clinical results over and above those seen with silver sol. See www.silverhealthinstitute.com for further information.

Ecuador

Deep in the jungles of southeastern Ecuador, el Oriente, is a land that is home to the Shuar tribal peoples. While Ecuador has roughly 10% of its population from European extraction, about 90% are indigenous peoples of approximately 27 different tribes across the nation. Some of these are high mountain peoples, such as the Quichua of the Andes, while others are Amazonian jungle peoples. Unfortunately, the economic reality is inverted in Ecuador, as roughly 90% of the wealth of the nation is in the hands of the minority and only 10% of the wealth is in the hands of the majority indigenous peoples. Such a situation leads to extreme poverty, subsistence living and farming, and often lack of basic needs, including medical care.

The Shuar of el Oriente were headhunters until a generation ago. Now, many live in government protected reservations, much as is seen with many Native American tribal peoples. Yet, without casino gaming, oil and gas and other economic resources as are now going to American Native peoples, this is not the case in Ecuador.

GMP has served in Ecuador for 14 years, first high in the Andes at elevations of 9,000 to 12,000 feet, home of the beautiful Quichua peoples. For the last three years, GMP served the Shuar in the cool, dry and gorgeous jungles of southeast Ecuador. In our project in June 2010, a small boy came to the clinic with a laceration on his foot. While this may be a simple problem for many in North America, lack of health education, even including basic washing and asepsis, is often unknown. His infection demonstrated a nasty wound with the redness of cellulitis around the laceration. Thorough cleaning of the wound was made and silver gel, donated to GMP by Muvezi Health Projects Society of Canada, was applied. This was to be reapplied 2-3 times per day, in addition to one tablespoon of liquid silver twice daily. Based on follow-up reports, the boy experienced clearing of the wound much more rapidly than expected, even from the best of conventional medical care.

Other applications of silver on our projects in Ecuador have included topical wound infections as well as eye, ear and nasal purulent infections as well as other upper respiratory infections. The solution is not painful and has been highly effective when used in place of optic (eye) or otic (ear) antibiotic solutions, such as ciprofloxacin or gentamycin drops.

Nepal

Kathmandu sits on a high plane, approximately 4,200 feet above sea level, surrounded by a ring of hills at 8,000 to 12,000 feet high. On a clear day, free from the usual pollution, the Himalaya show their snowy splendor, reaching 18,000 to 29,035 feet, the southern slopes of Mt. Everest (Sagarmatha to the Nepali, Mother Goddess of the Universe).

GMP has served in over 24 missions to Nepal in the last 16 years. On one project to Nepal, a small girl presented with matting and drainage from her eyes. These eye infections are highly contagious even in the USA, and can spread to all in a family members living in small village homes very rapidly.

Using a small plastic dropper, silver is dropped into both eyes, 2-3 drops each, 2-3 times per day. As with external ear infections, we have seen the silver drops remedy these infections, typically within 24 hours. Further, the drops do not sting the eyes or the ears and thus they are well tolerated and received.

We have also had many patients do well clinically in Nepal with silver for vaginal and urinary complaints, using the solution both orally and topically (topical gel for vaginal inflammation or infections). Additionally, our team even reports recent successes with silver gel for psoriasis that was resistant to conventional care.

Beyond these common conditions, we have used silver gel with leprosy patients for their very serious wounds that develop due to sensory and motor nerve defects which accompany this horrible disease. Silver used topically as the gel or as the solution soaking a gauze on the lesion, as well as oral silver, has demonstrated tissue wound healing that often is better than that seen with conventional antibiotic and skin wound care.

Conclusions

Structured Silver solution and gel have proven to be very effective therapeutic agents for both the mission health camps and for the health of the team as it travels. The wide range of anti-bacterial, anti-viral, anti-parasitic and anti-fungal properties make it useful for treating many clinical infections. As it is non-painful and can be used orally as well as on any body surface or in any body opening, there is wide acceptance for use by patients.

Corporations with international workers and mission organizational leaders should seriously consider the use of silver as the first line of defense for their teams and for their patients. At times, if the silver has not satisfactorily resolved a clinical problem quickly, it may be used in conjunction with other pharmaceuticals with no conflict or harm. As this is an emerging technology that is not yet widely known, all corporations with international workers and mission organizational leaders are encouraged to share the information about Structured Silver and its many uses so that their employees, consultants and volunteers may be fully informed as to options for their own health as well as that of those they will treat on mission projects.

How to purchase the new Structured Silver

Further information regarding Structured Silver may be found at www.silverhealthinstitute.com. For lay consumers, Thank You Silver is the finest available in Structured Silver for purchases available to the public. Please visit www.ThankYouSilver.com for purchase; be sure to use the DISCOUNT CODE "54321" for discounts on your purchases.

For professionals, please contact www.TravelDoc.info for an application to purchase pH Structured Silver for your practice at wholesale pricing. Professionals include physicians, surgeons, osteopaths, dentists, chiropractors, pharmacists, naturopaths, doctors of oriental medicine, veterinarians, physician assistants, nurse practitioners, physical therapists, occupational therapists and physical therapy assistants.

Chapter 3
Activated Charcoal for Travel

One of the truly exciting and natural remedies in addition to Structured Silver is so deceptively ordinary at first appearance and, to many, even appears "dirty". Yet, charcoal, specifically *activated charcoal,* possesses extraordinary properties that may help us to clear toxins, fight microbial infections and other significant health-producing effects. Clearly, activated charcoal will be the second remedy in this author's travel kit, along with Structured Silver.

Ancient history records the use of charcoal by numerous civilizations for thousands of years, with the first recorded use in 3750 B.C. as fuel to smelt ores since charcoal burns much hotter than wood. Charcoal has numerous applications in industry, food science, toxicology, space travel and has been listed for its therapeutic values in the medical literature of its day by the Egyptians as early as 1500 B.C., Hippocrates circa 400 B.C. and Pliny the Elder in 50 A.D. The recommendations in medical literature continue to Claudius Galen of the second century A.D., perhaps Rome's most famous physician of his day and continuing into this current era.

Charcoal is the blackened residual of burning wood and other products without complete consumption of the product itself. For the purposes of medicinal care, hardwoods, coconut shells and bones are the most common starting materials. Commercial, medical or food-grade charcoal is called activated charcoal. Activated charcoal is listed by the USA Federal Drug Administration (FDA) as a Class 1, "safe and effective" agent to treat for acute poisoning. In fact, activated charcoal is present in essentially every emergency room in the country for its effectiveness in *adsorbing* the poisons and thus decreasing the potential loss of life and health, yet without adverse side effects.

Activated charcoal is further processed by exposing the source material to gas or to oxygen or steam at extremely high temperatures, resulting in a carbonization or oxidation process wherein the material is micro-porous, with pores measuring only 1 micron in high quality activated charcoal. Due to this micro-porosity, one gram (1/4th of a tablespoon) will have a surface area of 500 – 1500+ m^{-2}, as determined by gas adsorption. Adsorption, rather than absorption is the process of action. A hand towel is able to *absorb* water spilled on the kitchen sink as the water permeates the dry towel. On the other hand, charcoal *adsorbs* gases and liquids, a process whereby gases, liquids or dissolved solids are adhered to the micro-pore structure of the charcoal. This occurs due to the structural framework and the resultant Van der Waal's forces. Charcoal demonstrates the remarkable varying structure of carbon atoms as is seen in such diversity of carbon as that soft carbon in the graphite of a pencil compared to the incredible hardness and density of a diamond. Both, as well as charcoal, contain simply carbon in different form and structure.

Medicinal activated charcoal is available in powder, tablets, capsules, even toothpaste, and can be used internally and topically for a diverse set of clinical situations. As mentioned previously, charcoal adsorbs enormous quantities of toxins and poisons per given quantity of charcoal, yet its uses extend far beyond poisoning and toxicities. A study published in the British medical journal, The Lancet, reported significant reductions of total cholesterol by 25%, LDL by 41% and a doubling of the

HDL/LDL (high density lipoprotein/low density lipoprotein) ratio. This was presented in patients who took two tablespoons of activated charcoal three times daily for four weeks only!

Activated charcoal adsorbs and/or inactivates bacteria, viruses, fungi and parasites have each been demonstrated to in laboratory (in vitro) or live (in vivo) research. Charcoal filters are used in many portable and industrial water treatment devices and are readily available in lightweight, portable containers. Clinical applications are lengthy and a sampling is included in Tables 3.1, 3.2 and 3.3.

Clinical applications for activated charcoal

Table 3.1 Gastrointestinal applications, activated charcoal

Appendicitis
Colic
Constipation
Crohn's Disease
Diarrhea/ Dysentery
Duodenal ulcers
Dyspepsia
Flatulence
Food poisoning
Gallstones
Halitosis (bad breath)
Hemorrhoid
Hepatitis
Hypercholesterolemia
Indigestion
Intestinal worms
Jaundice
Nausea
Pancreatitis

Table 3.2 Infectious applications for activated charcoal

Abscesses/Boils
Candidiasis
Cholera
Conjunctivitis (Pink Eye)
Decubitus ulcers (bed/pressure sores)
Dental abscess
Diphtheria
Foot ulcers
Herpes labialis (cold sores)
HIV-1
Otitis (ear infection)
Pharyngitis (sore throat)
Smallpox
Tetanus
Tuberculosis
Typhoid
Urinary Tract Infection (UTI)

Table 3.3 General applications for activated charcoal

Gout
Hemostasis (blood coagulation)
Insect bites/stings
Plant fertilizer
Plant insecticide
Prostatitis
Scorpion stings
Spider bites
Snake bites
Water treatment
* NOTE: *Consultation with a competent healthcare professional is appropriate for all infectious illnesses. Do NOT delay consultation even while you are using activated charcoal.*

Plant and other poisons or medications neutralized by activated charcoal

Plant poisonings neutralized by activated charcoal include an extensive list seen in Table 3.4. In these cases, activated charcoal poultices may be applied topically, as in the case of poison ivy or stinging nettle when there is a skin response, or internally when these plants are internally consumed.

Activated charcoal can also adsorb and neutralize various pharmaceutical medications. In this case, the clinical effect of one needing these medications would likely be diminished. If however, there is an overdose of the medications, activated charcoal is often used in emergency departments across the nation for this type of ingestion. Likely a surprise to many physicians and nurses in emergency settings, studies have demonstrated that *inducing of vomiting does not further decrease the poison risk beyond the use of the activated charcoal* in appropriate quantities alone. Medications that will likely be adsorbed and neutralized include fluoxetine (Prozac®), acetaminophen (Tylenol®), as well as morphine, caffeine, nicotine and theobromine.

For poisons and chemicals, it is critical to NEVER induce vomiting when a caustic or corrosive poison has been consumed. Further, as studies have demonstrated that inducing of vomiting dose *not* further decrease the poison risk beyond the use of appropriate quantities of activated charcoal alone, as just noted above. When the amount of poison consumed is unknown, a general rule of activated charcoal antidote would be approximately 1 gram of activated charcoal per 1 kg. of body weight, or roughly ½ gram activated charcoal per 1 pound of body weight. While this is a generally guideline for emergency treatment, *ALL poisoning patients should be cared for by competent emergency healthcare providers as soon as available.*

In a critical situation without the availability of emergency medical services and with an unconscious patient, activated charcoal should NOT be forced down the patient's mouth, for fear of aspiration or spilling into the lungs. Instead, a poultice of activated charcoal may be placed on the skin over the liver and perhaps the kidneys as well, and there have been reports that this neutralized the ingested poison. Again, *ALL poisoning patients should be cared for by competent emergency healthcare providers as soon as available.*

Table 3.4 Botanical poisons neutralized by activated charcoal

Alder
Autumn crocus
Azalea
Black nightshade
Bryony
Buckthorn berry
Christmas rose
Daphne
Deadly nightshade
Foxglove
Hemlock
Holly berry
Honeysuckle berry
Jerusalem cherry
Laburnum
Lily of the Valley

Table 3.4 Botanical poisons neutralized by activated charcoal, (continued)

Mistletoe
Monk's Hood
Oleander
Poison ivy
Poison oak
Poison sumac
Privet Berry
Rhodendron
Savin juniper
Spindle tree berry
Thorn apple
Woody nightshade
Yew

Contraindications to activated charcoal

The only contraindications appear to be that sufficient water be taken orally when using charcoal for constipation, and also in the treatment of variegate porphyria, a rare skin disease.

While there is some concern for the possibility of a tattooing effect when applying charcoal on open wounds, this does not generally seem to be an issue, and should be minimized if the charcoal is placed with a barrier such as a moist gauze, muslin cloth or paper towel against the wound surface.

How to make an activated charcoal poultice

Activated charcoal poultices are easy to make and have proven beneficial for many topical illnesses as well as internal illnesses. At its most easy application, pure charcoal powder may be sprinkled on topical wounds, including skin ulcers, abrasions, cuts, decubitus ulcers (bed/pressure sores) and others. Activated charcoal may be applied with a gauze, muslin cloth or paper towel to provide a barrier between the activated charcoal powder and the topical surface. Using this technique, the poultice may also be applied over the closed eyelids for eye infections, on the ears for otitis, in the nose for hemostasis of epistaxis (stopping a nosebleed) and on the skin for ant bites, bee/wasp stings, scorpion stings, spider bites, snakebites and topical eruptions as from poison ivy, oak or sumac. *Clearly, use of activated charcoal in these situations does not replace consultation with a competent healthcare professional.*

It is imperative that the activated charcoal poultice be moistened enough that the dressing will *remain moist* for 10-12 hours while in place. A dry poultice will not adsorb and neutralize the intended target. A great poultice may be made from equal parts of powdered activated charcoal and ground flax seed, or alternately with therapeutic clay such as Bentonite or Zeolite.

For example, mix equal parts of powdered activated charcoal and ground flax seed. It is wise to grind flax seed in a blender prior to travel as part of an emergency kit. With the dry mix, add water to make a wet, yet not runny, mixture. Use a gauze, muslin cloth or paper towel large enough to cover the area to be treated and for approximately 1-2" beyond. Be sure the poultice is moist; flaxseed poultices typically retain the moisture well even throughout the night. Cover the poultice with plastic, even Saran Wrap will do. Cover the entire poultice with an elastic bandage to keep in place throughout the day or night until it is changed. Typically replace the poultice twice each 2 hours and discard the used poultice as it will have adsorbed toxins and microbes and is not reusable.

Chapter 4
Botanical/Herbal Remedies for Travel

The term "herb" is broadly defined as a non-woody plant that dies down to the ground after flowering. The term "botanical" is a more general description of flora, although common interpretation describes any plant used for medicinal therapy, nutritional value or food seasoning or dyeing (coloring). As with acupuncture, homeopathy and other natural therapeutics, the use of botanicals may be encountered in travels as a part of the indigenous culture and healthcare. Botanicals are often prepared as teas or infusions, with the plant's soft portions placed in a pot and covered by boiling water to create a supernatant. Herbal decoctions are traditionally prepared in special earthen crocks or in containers of stainless steel, ceramic or enamel by contemporary practitioners, specifically avoiding aluminum and alloy metal pots. The herb is placed in the container and covered with cold water that is then boiled, covered and simmered.

Travelers may encounter a botanical/herbal remedy dispensed as a poultice, botanical liniment, ointment or oil to be applied to the skin. Alternately, many modern herbalists utilize capsule forms for ease of administration. Combinations of several herbs are often more effective than a single herb, and common formulae have been recorded worldwide for centuries. Appropriate application or prescription of botanical products rarely leads to toxicity or adverse reactions, although such are possible if botanicals are used excessively or carelessly, or if the raw products are tainted through poor farming or manufacturing processes.

Botanical healing may rightly be considered original healing and the subject of many home remedies that have been effective for primitive and sophisticated peoples alike. Hippocrates' admonition, "Let your food be medicine and your medicine be food," would serve us well in our contemporary lives. Many physicians have recited the Hippocratic Oath upon conferring their Medical Degree and know well another of his great lines, *"Primum non nocerum"* (First do no harm). Botanical preparations are often a superb way to prepare for and to respond to the challenges of travel.

The Bible tells us how God has placed plants on the earth for our use and to promote and enjoy good health.

Ezekiel 47:12

Fruit trees of all kinds will grow on both banks of the river. Their leaves will not wither, nor will their fruit fail. Every month they will bear fruit, because the water from the sanctuary flows to them. Their fruit will serve for food and their leaves for healing.

Poultices, salves, tinctures, teas and other forms of botanical and herbal products have been used for millennia for preserving and regaining health. Some of the more common ailments experienced during travel are readily and ably resolved by botanical and herbal remedies without the common side effects of usual pharmaceutical preparations. Even today, scientists and medical anthropologists continue to make new botanical discoveries for health in jungles, deserts and other lands worldwide.

While most integrative physicians recognize that botanical/herbal remedies are typically safer and with less side effects (even with side benefits!) than conventional pharmaceutical prescription or over-the-counter remedies, it is still important to be cautious and to know with certainty what a particular botanical remedy is before taking it. Poisonous or tainted botanical products are sold globally, so a reputable and reliable source for your botanical remedies is critical.

Common botanical/herbal remedies for travel

How to use botanical/herbal remedies for travel

Botanical and herbal remedies are readily available through online Internet sources as well as numerous health stores. Through these sources, botanicals are commonly in dried, loose-leaf form to make teas and poultices, as tinctures and commonly as single or combination products in capsules. Many will find the tinctures and capsules to be the easiest to carry on travel.

Based on the particular clinical need, as are highlighted in the sections below, one is able to choose their botanical selection and then take orally as a tea, tincture or capsule or topically as a poultice. Please also see Chapter 8 for a concise list of 12 botanical/herbal products to consider for your botanical/herbal travel first aid kit. The recommended amount of botanical/herbal products should be listed on the package or container purchased.

Prevention/immunization

It is always advisable to begin travel well and healthy. This should include consideration in the days to months ahead of travel to give the best chance of safe and well travel. Certain botanicals are useful to enhance the immune system and act as a general tonic.

Teas, capsules and powdered preparations that promote health and wellness in general are often available with multiple botanicals combined. These may commonly include Gingko biloba, American or Asian ginseng (*Panax quinquefolius or Panax ginseng*), echinacea (*Echinacea various species*), evening primrose (*Oenothera biennis*), garlic (*Allium sativum*), Gotu kola (*Centella asiatica*), milk thistle (*Sylibum marianum*), peppermint (*Mentha piperita*), parslane (*Portulaca oleracea*), thyme (*Thymus vulgaris*), chamomile (*Matricaria recutita*) and horsetail (*Equisetium arvense*).

Table 4.1 Botanical remedies for travel prevention

American ginseng
Asian ginseng
Chamomile
Echinacea
Evening Primrose
Garlic
Gingko biloba
Gotu kola
Horsetail
Milk thistle
Parslane
Peppermint
Thyme

Chinese botanical/herbal combinations are often found as "patent" herbal preparations, including Kang Ning Wan (also known as Coix Formula, consisting of coix, angelica, notopterygium, ledebouriella, atractylodes, cinnamomum, aconite, ligusticum, siegesbeckia, chaenomelis and poria). Coix Formula is well known to provide relief for motion sickness, food poisoning, excessive eating and drinking alcohol, nausea, headache, vomiting, diarrhea or constipation, gastrointestinal cramping and generalized pain.

The above botanicals, and certainly others, provide anti-oxidant, anti-aging and anti-inflammatory effects and may help promote better energy, clearer thinking, better mood and emotions, enhanced hormonal levels and immune support.

Jet lag /travel fatigue

St. John's Wort (*Hypericum perfolatum*) is a common over-the-counter remedy that is one of the most widely used botanicals in Europe for decades. St. John's Wort, named for its flowering on St. John's Day (June 24) and *wort* as the Old English word for plant, contains the compound hypericum, which has shown significant improvement for anxiety, depression and feelings of worthlessness in clinical studies. Some studies have also shown beneficial effects to improve sleep quality. Once thought to be due primarily do its MAO (Mono Amine Oxidase Inhibitor) effect, studies now indicate that there are more compounds and the combination of these gives good clinical effect with less to no side effects. *This botanical is NOT advised for pregnancy.*

Lemon balm or Melissa (*Melissa officinalis*) is also recommended by the German Commission E, both as a sedative and to soothe the stomach. Active compounds include terpenes, which are also found in juniper, ginger, basil and clove, although none of these has the reputation as a bedtime herb as lemon balm.

Valerian Root (*Valerian officinalis*), a third botanical endorsed by the German Commission E for promotion of

Table 4.2 Botanical remedies for jet lag/travel fatigue

Chamomile
Lavender
Lemon balm/Melissa
Passion flower
Rooibos
St. John's Wort
Valerian root

sleep is commonly taken as a tea, although capsules may be easier for travel. It has been recommended for anxiety, restlessness and nervousness as well. More than 80 over-the-counter sleeping aids in the United Kingdom contain Valerian Root, and the common hangover feeling often associated with prescription anxiety and sleep medications is not prevalent with this plant remedy.

Lavender (*Lavandula, various species*) is commonly used in massage therapy clinics in the massage oil or diffused into the air to promote relaxation and rest as well as to reduce irritability. Beware, however, as some species of lavender are actually stimulating, notably Spanish Lavender.

Passionflower (*Passiflora incarnata*) is a mild sedative, included in over 40 over-the-counter sleep preparations in the UK. In spite of extensive use worldwide for centuries to treat nervous tension, anxiety and insomnia, the US FDA has not approved this botanical remedy.

Chamomile (*Matricaria recutita*) tea has been used as a bedtime tea for centuries. The chemical, apigenin, has demonstrated to be one of the most effective sedative botanical compounds.

Rooibos (*Aspalathus linearis*) is a shrubby African legume that is a favorite for bedtime tea among many in South Africa. Its popularity has spread and is usually now available in the US as a tea. In addition to promoting sleep, it has been used to calm the digestive tract, reduce nervous tension and is generally considered safe enough to give to infants.

Cough/cold/flu

Echinacea, the Mountain Daisy or Coneflower, has perhaps received more attention, likely rightly so, in the lay health magazines and literature in the USA and abroad than any other single botanical. The Great Plains Indians of Native America have chewed Echinacea for centuries to treat colds, flu and other ailments. Naturopathic and integrative medical doctors alike have encouraged Echinacea for general immune support by nationally and internationally renowned practitioners.

Much research on Echinacea has been performed, with perhaps the greatest collection in German medical literature. Echinacea increases a chemical in the body called properdin, which activates part of the immune system responsible for increasing defense against viruses and bacteria. Echinacea extracts have demonstrated anti-viral activity against influenza, herpes and other viruses.

Garlic (*Allium sativum*) contains the chemical allicin, one of the plant kingdom's most potent, broad-spectrum antibiotics. Additionally, ginger (*Zingiber officinale*) contains nearly a dozen anti-viral compounds, including sesquiterpenes that have specific action against the most common family of cold viruses, known as rhinoviruses. Other compounds include gingerols and shogaols, known to relieve pain and fever, suppress coughing and mildly sedate to encourage rest. Onion (*Allium cepa*) is closely related to garlic and has similar anti-viral activities.

Citrus fruits and other plants containing Vitamin C are important as a part of our diets, or as supplemented to prevent cold symptoms. Amazonian fruit camu-camu (*Myrciaria dubia*) has the world's highest Vitamin C content and other good sources include acerola, bell peppers, cantaloupe and pineapple.

Elderberry (*Sambucus nigra*) is an herb containing two compounds that are active against influenza viruses and also prevents the virus from invading the respiratory tract cells. Israeli patented drug Sambucol® contains elderberry and has demonstrated anti-viral activity in preliminary trials against Epstein-Barr virus, herpes and HIV.

Forsythia (*Forsythia suspense*) and honeysuckle (*Lonicera japonica*) are common Chinese traditional approaches to treating colds and flu. They, too, demonstrate anti-viral properties in research.

Anise (*Pimpinella anisum*) is recognized by the German Commission E as an expectorant, to thin mucus and rid the phlegm. Anise also has demonstrated anti-viral properties in larger doses.

Ephedra (*Ephedra sinica*) is known as Ma Huang in Traditional Chinese Medicine, and has long been used as a potent decongestant. Ephedra's chemicals, ephedrine and pseudoephedrine, dilate bronchial airways. Caution is important as the compounds in Ephedra may also lead to elevating blood pressure, insomnia and jitteriness. The US FDA has placed restrictions on the distribution of these due to occasional deaths, especially with overuse.

Table 4.3 Botanical remedies for cough/cold/flu

Anise
Citrus fruits:
> Acerola
> Bell peppers
> Camu camu
> Cantaloupe
> Grapefruit
> Kumquat
> Lemon
> Lime
> Orange
> Nectarine
> Pineapple
> Tangerine

Elderberry
Ephedra/Ma Huang
Forsythia
Goldenseal
Licorice
Marsh mallow
Serieka snakeroot
Slippery elm
watercress

Other botanical considerations may include goldenseal (*Hydratis canadensis*), licorice (*Glycyrrhiza glabra*), marsh mallow (*Althaea officinalis*), Seneka Snakeroot (*Polygala senega*), Slippery Elm (*Ulmus rubra*) and watercress (*Nasturtium officinale*).

Diarrhea/dysentery or vomiting/hangover

While using botanicals or any other remedy for diarrhea, it is critical to continue to maintain adequate hydration through oral, and intravenous means, if necessary. The primary medical risk of common diarrhea still remains dehydration.

Commonly travelers will use a pharmaceutical such as Lomotil® (diphenoxylate/atropine), Immodium® (loperamide), or similar to stop diarrhea. While this may be helpful or necessary while a person is en route on planes, trains or other public transport, it is important to remember that most microbes that cause diarrhea *need to be cleared from the intestinal tract*. This means that while diarrhea can be stressful and unpleasant, it is in fact the body's process for eliminating the offending agent. To use the anti-diarrheal agents to stop or slow the bowel movements, this author generally recommends against their use unless necessitated for travel, then to stop the pharmaceutical and allow the body to expel the offenders as soon as is possible.

Botanicals may help to quiet the intestinal tract, though not typically as aggressively as pharmaceutical agents. A significant relief from cramping may allow one to continue to eliminate the agent in a more controlled fashion and reach recovery faster overall.

Most botanicals that help to calm diarrhea have the compounds tannin, pectin and/or mucilage. Tannins have an astringent action that decreases intestinal inflammation. Pectin is a soluble fiber that adds bulk to the stool and soothes the gut. Pectin is the "pectate" in the over-the-counter anti-diarrheal medicine Kaopectate®. Mucilage sooths the digestive tract and adds bulk to the stool by absorbing water and decreasing swelling.

Agrimony (*Agrimonia eupatoria*) contains high amounts of tannin and is Commission E endorsed for common diarrhea. Apple (*Malus domestica*) pulp is high in pectin, which has a property noted as "amphoteric". This means that it will act as a remedy for diarrhea and also it will help with constipation because of its action as a stool softener.

Bilberry and blueberry (*Vaccinium, various species*) are rich in both pectin and tannins and thus offer relief for common diarrhea. Blackberry and raspberry (*Rubus, various species*) are also both high in tannins and are often effective for common diarrhea.

Carob (*Ceratonia siliqua*) powder has been shown in studies to reduce diarrhea duration by as much as fifty percent in children with bacterial or viral diarrhea.

Carrots (*Daucus carota*) are good choices for adults or infants for diarrhea. Cooked carrots soothe the digestive tract, decrease diarrhea and provide vitamins and minerals often lost during sickness.
Fenugreek (*Trigonella foenum-graecum*) seed contain up to 50 percent mucilage. Thus, they swell in the gut to relieve diarrhea and also soften the stool, so also an amphoteric, like apple. Portions should be limited to limit the potential for gut irritability that may be experienced with too large a dose.

Oak (*Quercus, various species*) is recommended by the German Commission E for diarrhea by making a tea of 2 teaspoons of dried oak bark.

Psyllium (*Plantago ovata*) is often known for its use in relieving constipation, however, as another amphoteric, it also has a high mucilage content that makes it useful for treating diarrhea. Caution is advised with this botanical that if allergic symptoms arise after one use, this is not to be used further.

Table 4.4 Botanical remedies for diarrhea/dysentery or vomiting/hangover

Agrimony
Apple
Bilberry
Blackberry
Blueberry
Carob
Carrots
Fenugreek
Oak
Psyllium
Raspberry

Pain/trauma

It is critically important to have proper evaluation by a competent health care provider for issues that present with pain that is anything beyond the ordinary experience for the traveler. With this in mind, there are a number of botanicals that should be considered for pain issues on travel.

Aloe (*Aloe vera*) has been used since ancient times to treat burns and other wounds and trauma. By slitting the succulent plant's fat, leathery leaves, the gel is easily obtained and applied topically, or may be taken internally. Aloe has anti-bacterial and ant-fungal properties and is anti-inflammatory as well.

Arnica (*Arnica Montana*), or coneflower, is well recognized for its efficacy to treat trauma, bruises, swelling and other wounds. It may be used botanically or homeopathically with great success in most situations.

The German Commission E recommends Calendula (*Calendula officinalis*) for reducing inflammation and promoting wound healing. It has immune-enhancing properties and is anti-bacterial and anti-viral. Calendula may be taken internally as a tea or applied topically as a poultice of the dry petals and is readily available as a topical cream. Rubbing the flower on a bee or wasp sting will likely take care of both pain and swelling.

Clove (*Syzygium aromaticus*) has been recognized for its usefulness for dental pain in folk medicine and this is confirmed by the German Commission E. Clove oil is applied directly to the gum and tooth involved.

Evening primrose (*Oenothera biennis*) is rich in the amino acid tryptophan. Studies have demonstrated that tryptophan supplements are effective in relieving pain of acute and chronic conditions. While the oil has been often recommended in some circles, much of the tryptophan is lost in the oil-extraction process; so powdered seeds should be a better choice.

Ginger (*Zingiber officinale*) studies have shown ginger to be a highly effective pain reliever, using 2-4 teaspoons of powdered ginger daily. Further, ginger may be applied to painful areas topically, such as with hot ginger compresses for abdominal cramps, headache or joint pain.

Kava kava (*Piper methysticum*) is a tropical herb that has demonstrated analgesic effectiveness comparable to aspirin. Described as a narcotic, kava kava is recognized to be non-addictive. Chewing the leaves will lead to numbness of the mouth, and therefore useful for dental pain, canker sores and sore throat.

Peppermint (*Mentha piperita*) contains menthol, which has anesthetic effects. Studies have demonstrated significant pain relieving effects using peppermint. However, as peppermint oil is typically very concentrated, mix a few drops in a tablespoon of coconut or olive oil to decrease the potential to irritate the skin. Never drink peppermint oil, as a small amount can be toxic.

Red pepper (*Capsicum, various species*) has become a popular natural choice for pain therapy in the last decade or two, even in over-the-counter or pharmaceutical preparations. Pain-relieving compounds called salicylates, similar to salicins, are the botanical equivalent of aspirin. Additionally, the red peppers contain capsaicin, a compound that stimulates the body's natural endorphins, and also depleting the pain transmitter, Substance P. *When used topically, these preparations should be used repeatedly each day to keep the Substance P depleted.* Also, be sure to wash your hands thoroughly after applying the creams, so as not to accidentally place it in the eyes. Finally, as some are sensitive to Capsicum creams, it is wise to use a small portion on a limited area first, to determine that it will be tolerated, and to discontinue use if it leads to skin irritation.

Turmeric (*Curcuma longa*) is found in curries and has long been a staple of South Asian cuisine. It has some of the most potent botanical anti-inflammatory properties known. Turmeric has gained in recognition and popularity recently and is available widely in health food stores and pharmacies.

Willow bark (*Salix, various species*) contains salicin, from which aspirin was derived just over 100 years ago. Commission E endorsed, willow may provide relief for a wide variety of pains. Beware: willow should be avoided by those who are allergic to aspirin compounds and do NOT give willow or similar products or aspirin to young children who have a viral syndrome as the risk of Reye's Syndrome, hepato-encephalopathy, may develop.

Table 4.5 Botanical remedies for pain/trauma

Arnica Montana
Clove
Evening primrose
Ginger
Kava kava
Peppermint
Red pepper
Turmeric
Willow

Chinese botanical/herbal combinations are long-held in regard for efficacy of pain and trauma, including Zheng Gu Shui. This herbal combination lists camphor 5.6% and menthol 5.6% as active ingredients and bushy knotweed, camphor wood extract, Angelica root, Moghania root, Zedoary rhizome and ginseng root, as inactive ingredients. Many have found this to be wonderful for sprains, strains, bruises, muscle pain and arthritis pain.

Frostbite or heat exhaustion/sunstroke

Ginkgo biloba should be considered as a botanical approach to managing frostbite, or chilblains. Containing numerous compounds including terpenes, flavones, proanthocyanidins, ginkgolides and others, the leaves have demonstrated the ability to improve arterial and venous circulation, especially in the brain, eyes, ears and limbs. Since the circulatory benefits were discovered in the 1960s, ginkgo has been used as a vasodilator and also has been shown to scavenge free radicals, perhaps the mechanism for its protective effect on vascular walls. Common dosages are 50 mg up to three times daily.

Aloe (*Aloe vera*) has been used since ancient times to treat burns and other wounds and trauma. As aloe is known to increase circulation of damaged tissue, it is well indicated for frostbite.

Common oak (*Quercus rubor*), with its astringent properties, may be applied topically as a poultice of the leaves, bark and acorns or as a tea or capsule. Lungwort (*Pulmonaria officinalis*), commonly known in French as "the cardia herb" has been recognized for benefit for frostbite. Black walnut (*Juglans nigra*) as well has been listed as a remedy for frostbite in various publications.

Table 4.6 Botanical remedies for frostbite or heat exhaustion/sunstroke

Frostbite

Aloe vera
Black walnut
Common oak
Ginkgo biloba
Lungwort

Heat exhaustion/sunstroke

Black mulberry
Ginseng, American
Ginseng, Siberian
Passionflower
Peppermint

Sunstroke and overheating may be addressed with a variety of botanicals to cool the body and help to dispel excess heat.

American ginseng (*Panax quinquefolium*) or Siberian ginseng (*Eleutherococcus senticosus*) are also noted for efficacy in heat exhaustion, prepared as a tea. Peppermint (*Mentha piperata*) should be considered as a cool forehead compress or orally. Black mulberry *(Morus nigra)* may be beneficial, prepared as a tea. Passionflower (*Passiflora incarnata)* is also noted for clinical benefits to sunstroke and heat exhaustion.

Most importantly, adequate hydration and mineral replacement are critical for anyone suffering from heat exhaustion, commonly associated with dehydration. A good general rule is to consume one quart or liter of water for each 50 pounds of body weight daily. Beyond this, additional water may be necessary if strenuous activity is engaged.

New horizons for botanical health

Haus Bioceuticals (see Resources) has developed new, novel botanical products that are very promising for a variety of indications. Botanical remedies include topical cream or liquid that have remarkable effects clinically on eczema, psoriasis, diabetic ulcers and bedsores. Additionally, their novel formulation of curcumin leads to 500-1000s of times higher blood levels and may prove very important for anti-inflammatory considerations, arthritis and even cancers. More products and developments are underway and this should prove to be a very useful resource for botanical health and wellness.

Chapter 5
Homeopathic Remedies for Travel

Dr. Samuel Hahnemann was a German medical physician who developed a novel system of healing therapeutics in the late 1700s. Indeed, the practice of classical homeopathy is a highly specialized field of medicine and requires medical doctors, naturopathic physicians and others to study for years, just as with any other medical or healthcare specialty. Yet, a variety of contemporary homeopathic remedies may be reasonably assessable to the general public that may help protect from or resolve various ailments commonly experienced with travel.

Hahnemann theorized that substances, which led to various symptoms in their gross presence, could potentially stimulate the body to adjust and heal various symptoms with a very small amount of the same substances. Because the remedies in homeopathic medicine are diluted to extremely miniscule levels, many conventional allopathic physicians reject the theories and practice completely. Many homeopathic remedies are diluted and also *succussed* or activated, a process called *potentized* or *dynamized* in homeopathy to a level below Avagadro's Number (6.02×10^{-23} particles/mole of solution), that point of dilution at which no more of the original matter exists in solution.

This point of dilution is not a problem for homeopathy, as it is the *informational and energetic signature* or imprint upon the carrying liquid that affects the therapeutic benefits, not the physical substance. Centuries of homeopathic medicine have now passed and homeopathy has a strong footing in most of the world, with a unique exception lacking among American conventional medicine.

Homeopathic practitioners, while small and growing in number in the USA, are widely found across most of the globe.

In classic medical history, British physician Thomas Sydenham (1624-1689) is often recognized as the Father of Modern Clinical Medicine". His clinical method was based on very detailed observations of patients and the natural history of illness. Dr. Sydenham regarded illness as "an effort of nature, who strives with might and main to restore the health of the patient by the elimination of morbific matter". He introduced, for example, quinine (cinchona) for the treatment of ague (malaria) out of this precise and painstaking approach to patient evaluation. Interestingly, it was out of this work with quinine that Hahnemann first ventured into his homeopathic method.

What may be quite a surprise to many Americans is that many of the finest medical colleges in America were started as homeopathic medical colleges, such as Hahnemann in Philadelphia, PA. In 1900, it is estimated that 15% of physicians in the USA prescribed homeopathic remedies. Following the presentation of the Flexner Report to Congress in 1910, in an effort to eradicate "snake oil salesman" and other "unfounded" remedies, much of traditional healthcare, including homeopathy, was forced out of American medicine. In spite of the decades of pharmaceutical and surgical monopolies' activities on the regulatory boards and medical training institutions, valid Complementary and Alternative Medicine (CAM) practices have been slowly and steadily regaining proper placement back into American health care, though commonly uncovered by many or most private and government health insurance providers.

Some of the common "homeopathic" remedies available through health food stores or Internet sources to the public are actually "isopathic" remedies. For example, if a patient has a cold sore on their lip, *herpes labialis*, the isopathic remedy would be from a potentized remedy (diluted and succused, see above) of herpes simplex virus. However, from a homeopathic tradition, the "similimum" would be recognized that the herpes lesion on the lip is symptomatically very much like common poison ivy eruptions. Thus, the homeopathic remedy for the same lesion on the lip would be a potentized remedy or *rhus toxicondendron*, or poison ivy.

Both of these remedies, the homeopathic and the isopathic, may be highly effective remedies for the lesions and result in rapid clearing. The purpose here is to make the reader aware of a technical and important differences between true homeopathic remedies and what are often labeled as such in commercial sources.

Classical homeopathy utilizes only one agent or remedy at a time at only a single potency. Modern or complex homeopathy often utilizes multiple agents and each perhaps at multiple potencies. The rationale is that the body will resonate only with the agents and at the potencies that are needed to effect the cure or remediation of the illness and the others will simply be ignored since they do not resonate with the symptom or pathology. This debate has been longstanding and will surely continue in years ahead.

Homeopathic remedies commonly come in liquid that is dropped or sprayed under the tongue, small pellets or tablets, also placed under the tongue, or as topical liquids or creams and gels. Given the science and mechanisms of homeopathy, it is not necessary to use the topical for surface issues, and all conditions may commonly be treated with the sublingual forms.

Finally, before discussing some common travel issues that may well respond to homeopathic remedies commonly availably to the public without prescription, it is this author's belief that homeopathic remedies should not be take casually or for long term. *Consultation with a trained homeopathic physician should always be encouraged for long-term health intervention and continuation of therapy.*

Common homeopathic remedies for travel

How to use homeopathic remedies for travel

Homeopathic remedies are readily available through online Internet sources as well as numerous health stores. Through these sources, homeopathic remedies are commonly available for oral use as small pellets or as liquid drops or spays commonly used sublingually (under the tongue) and topically as creams or gels. All of these forms are easy to carry on travel.

Based on the particular clinical need, as are highlighted in the sections below, one is able to choose their homeopathic remedy selection and then take orally as pellets, drops or spray under the tongue or topically as a cream or gel. Please also see Chapter 8 for a concise list of 12 homeopathic remedies to consider for your homeopathic travel first aid kit. The recommended amount of homeopathic remedies may be listed on the package or container purchased.

Unless otherwise noted, for acute injuries and illnesses, most homeopathic preparations should be considered in 3X, 6X or 12X potency and given every 15-30 minutes immediately after injury or onset until symptoms improve. Typically 2-3 pellets or 2-3 drops of homeopathic liquid under the tongue are adequate. If no effect is noticed after 2-3 doses, the homeopathic selection should be reconsidered. Aconite 3X plus Bryonia 3X may be a trusted first aid remedy for nearly all acute illnesses, taking 5-10 drops under the tongue every 15 minutes for 2-3 hours, as needed.

Prevention/immunization

Some consider that immunizations are similar to homeopathic remedies in that with immunizations a particular bacteria or virus is given inactivated or in small quantity to stimulate the immune system to mount a response against the organism should it enter the body and the full presentation of the illness thus be prevented or attenuated. Many vaccines certainly contain a gross amount of the substance in question, often "attenuated" (inactivated) or made to be less virulent by genetic or chemical means.

Homeopathic approach, on the other hand, and more precisely "isopathic" approach, would be to take a truly potentized form of the bacteria or virus to prepare the immune system in the event of infection. In the case of homeopathic or isopathic remedies, there may be no actual physical presence of the organism remaining in solution, as described above. I this case, it is the energetic imprint on the solution that is felt to confer the benefit.

Homeopathic or isopathic remedies are available for many of the common and even rare transmittable illnesses, such as common flu or common cold, while others are available only through professional providers by highly reputable homeopathic labs (see Resources).

For first aid remedies, one should generally see a change in the clinical experience within an hour or two, and often work very promptly. If there is no response, one should likely change remedies. *Of course if symptoms persist, it is important to present to a competent healthcare practitioner.*

Jet lag /travel fatigue

Commonly experienced by many travelers while crossing multiple time zones and thereby being inserted into new time schedules, homeopathic remedies may provide significant relief.

Cocculus indica may be very useful for jet lag and to help restore the normal sleep/wake cycles in the new destination, as well as for motion sickness, as below.

Motion sickness/sea sickness

Cocculus indica and Tabacum are two leading homeopathic remedies for this common experience of motion or seasickness while on travel. Cocculus may also be very useful for jet lag and to help restore the normal sleep/wake cycles in the new destination, as noted above.

Cough/cold/flu

Many experience the onset of coughs, colds and/or flu due to travel and exposure to crowds along with the general weakening of the immune system when one is tired and fatigued from travel. Usually, pharyngitis is easily treated homeopathically. If a positive Strep culture is obtained, most will agree that antibiotic treatment of the Group A Beta Strep is important, as failure to do so could lead to future kidney (nephritis) and heart problems (carditis).

However, many upper respiratory infections are viral or of other bacteria and not of Strep.

Homeopathic remedies for pharyngitis include Belladonna, Hepar sulphurus, Ignatia, Mercuris vivus, Arsenicum ablum and others. Most effective may be the 30C potencies.

Coughs will also often respond well to homeopathic remedies. Commonly 30C potencies are recommended and doses taken each 8 hours. Bryonia alba is especially considered for colds that progress into the chest, and also for pleurisy. Causticum is indicated for dry, irritated coughs, often with a lot of mucus. Coccus cacti is indicated for coughs that come in paroxysms, or sudden, strong attacks.

Ipcacuanha is a main remedy for pertussis and also for COPD (Chronic Obstructive Pulmonary Disease). Kali bichromicum is indicated for a productive cough with very thick, green sputum. This is also heavily considered for purulent sinusitis. Kali carbonicum is for loose coughs with much mucus.

Phosphorus is a common remedy for recurrent coughs, hoarseness, yellow mucus and even pneumonia. Pulsatilla nigrans is perhaps the most common cough and cold remedy for children, especially for moist coughs that are worse while lying and at night. Sulfur is another common homeopathic remedy considered especially for children with night-time coughs. Arnica Montana is indicated when the whole body is sore with the cough.

Oscillococcinum is a commonly available flu remedy commonly used in homeopathy, best when taken in the first

Table 5.1 Homeopathic remedies for coughs/colds/flu

Aconite napellus
Arnica Montana
Arsenicum ablum
Baptisia
Belladonna
Bryonia alba
Causticum
Coccus cacti
Ferrum phosphoricum
Hepar sulphurus
Ignatia
Ipcacuanha
Kali bichromicum
Kali carbonicum
Mercuris vivus
Nux vomica
Oscillococcinum
Phosphorus
Pulsatilla nigrans
Rhus toxicodendron
Sulfur

24-48 hours of symptoms. Ferrum phosphoricum is also indicated for flu symptoms and is also best with taken in the first 24-48 hours of symptoms and Aconite napellus is recognized for benefit for colds and flu. Belladonna is also recognized for benefit for colds and flu and Nux vomica is to be considered especially when colds develop into influenza.

Arnica Montana, Bryonia alba and Rhus toxicodendron are to be considered, especially when flu is associated with severe aching. Arsenicum album, Baptisia, Bryonia alba and Nux vomica are flu remedies to consider when there are associated gastrointestinal symptoms of vomiting and/or diarrhea include.

Diarrhea/dysentery or vomiting/hangover

Food poisoning or food intoxication may lead to profuse vomiting and diarrhea while on travel. Certainly preparation and caution are best before consuming questionable food products. Ordering foods that are freshly and fully cooked, or where you can see them boiling or simmering offer some protection.

Arsenicum album may be the best overall homeopathic remedy for symptoms of diarrhea, dysentery, vomiting and hangover. China officianalis and Urtica urens, especially for shellfish poisoning are other homeopathic remedies to consider.

Table 5.2 Homeopathic remedies for diarrhea/dysentery or vomiting/hangover

Diarrhea/dysentery/vomiting

Arsenicum album
China officianalis
Urtica urens

Hangover

Arsenicum album
Nux vomica

Nux vomica is probably the most helpful, as well as prudent consumption, for those experiencing hangover from abuse of alcohol.

Maintaining hydration by oral or, if necessary by intravenous route, should be encouraged to prevent dehydration. As it is critical to staying well, repeating this is important. One should drink one quart or liter of clean water for each 50 pounds of body weight daily. More should be consumed if active or exercising.

Pain/trauma

Arnica Montana is likely the most widely recognized remedy for relieving pain from trauma. A North American native flower, the Mountain Daisy or Coneflower, this plant is often used in gross botanical preparations and also in homeopathic remedies. Some authors consider it useful in prophylactic considerations as well as symptomatically.

Staphysagria is another common homeopathic remedy for pain and trauma. Specifically it is recommended for trauma that is particularly intrusive to a person, where there is a strong sense of personal violation.

A commonly well-regarded complex homeopathic remedy is Traumeel® (see Resources, HeelUSA.com), indicated for sprains, strains, contusions, bruising, swelling and pain. Many German studies have demonstrated its efficacy. Additionally, the homeopathic complex Zeel® is intended to relieve joint pain associated with arthritis, as well as decreasing inflammation and joint stiffness, improving joint mobility. Other homeopathic pain/trauma remedies with their indications are included in Table 5.3.

Table 5.3 Homeopathic remedies for pain/trauma : indications

Arnica Montana : general pain remedy, swelling, prophylactic use

Aconitum napellus : eye injuries ("Arnica of the eye"), shock and great fear, natural disasters, accidents

Apis mellifica : swelling, burning, stinging pain

Arsenicum album : burns, especially 1st and 2nd degree

Bellis perennis : bruises, arthritis

Bryonia alba : cough, sprains worse with motion, mastitis (breast inflammation), fractured ribs

Calendula : abrasions, incised wounds

Cantharis : burns, especially 2nd and 3rd degree, urinary tract infections

Euptorium : fractures of bones

Hypericum perfollatum : sharp and shooting pains, especially nerve, compound fractures, corneal eye injuries, dental pain, injury to nerves and to coccyx, 1st and 2nd degree burns

Ledum palustre : penetrating injuries, bites and stings, splinters, black eye

Natrum sulphuricum : head injury

Rhus toxicodendron : sprains and strains, especially when worse in cold, damp weather, poison ivy, oak or sumac, general connective tissue swelling, arthritis

Ruta graveolans : tendon strains, Carpal Tunnel Syndrome, eyestrain

Staphysagria : incised wounds, urethral dilation

Symphytum : fractures of bones, eye pain

Urtical urens : stings, hives, burning and itching symptoms

Frostbite or heat exhaustion/sunstroke

While not commonly an experience in urban travel, wilderness and adventure or mission service travel may expose one to extreme cold and lead to frostbite. Homeopathic remedies may provide surprising benefit in frostbite to decrease pain and to spare tissue loss.

Agaricus is one of the main homeopathic remedies considered for frostbite. Apis mellifica, Pulsatilla and Rhus toxicodendron may also be useful to minimize pain and loss of tissue from the frostbite.

Heat exposure is likely a more common experience to travelers than is frostbite. Certainly, adequate hydration with safe, potable water is always important for travelers. Because it is so important, repeating intake as noted before is worthy. Daily clean water consumption should generally be 1 quart or liter for each 50 pounds of body weight.

Belladonna, Glonoinum and Natrum carbonicum are the main remedies for heat exhaustion and sunstroke.

Table 5.4 Homeopathic remedies for frostbite or heat exhaustion/sunstroke

Frostbite

Agaricus
Apis mellifica
Pulsatilla
Rhus toxicodendron

Table 5.4 Homeopathic remedies for frostbite or heat exhaustion/sunstroke, continued

Heat exhaustion/sunstroke

Belladonna
Glonoinum
Natrum carbonicum

Chapter 6
Essential Oil Remedies for Travel

Extracted through careful steam distillation and cold pressing, essential oils provide many opportunities for maintaining health and wellness for travel. Used around the world by various cultures for thousands of years, essential oils have health, cosmetic and emotional benefits. Essential oils are natural aromatic compounds found in the seeds, bark, stems, roots, flowers and other parts of plants. Highly fragrant, the aroma-therapeutic uses are only a part of the remarkable essential oil-rich benefits. Essential oils commonly deliver quick and potent clinical effects as the oils are much more powerful and effective than the dry herbal products. Essential oils may be diffused, inhaled, placed in baths, applied topically or taken internally for a variety of ailments. While essential oils are well absorbed, they do not build up in the body; they are excreted after yielding their remarkable benefits.

Likely the Egyptians were the first to use aromatic essential oils extensively in medical practice, beauty treatments, food preparations and religious ceremonies. Cinnamon, frankincense, myrrh and sandalwood were considered very valuable and at times were even exchanged for gold along the ancient trade routes. Others followed, including the ancient Greeks, Romans, Chinese, Indians and Persians. Essential oils were, used during the Dark Ages in Europe for their anti-bacterial and fragrant properties. Essential oils were used to maintain health, treat illness, and when all failed, to be included in the burial traditions around the globe.

French chemist, René-Maurice Gattefossé is credited with rediscovering the benefits of essential oils in recent times, having treated a badly burned hand with only pure lavender oil in 1937. Dr. Jean Valnet, a contemporary of Gattefossé, successfully treated injured soldiers in World War II, using therapeutic-grade essential oils. He continued his work with essential oils and became a renowned world leader in the development of aromatherapy practices.

Manufacture of essential oils is a highly specialized process and requires remarkable amounts of raw materials for distillation of the oils. For example, as many as 12,000 rose blossoms are required to distil 5 ml of essential rose oil, yet lavender only take 100 pounds of plant material to produce a pound of lavender essential oil. Beyond distillation, some citrus oils are extracted by compression and others by using solvents to extract the oils and then later removed from the final essential oil product.

Essential oils are thought to activate the brain's limbic system, its seat of emotions and memory; each different essential oil is felt to activate it differently. The smell of fragrant essences also stimulates various hormones and other metabolic processes. The olfactory (smell) responses to various fragrances have been documented extensively.

A wide range of emotional and physical wellness applications may be addressed with essential oils. The oils may be used individually or in complex blends, depending on user experience and desired benefits.

Many essential oils are high in anti-bacterial, anti-fungal and anti-viral properties. Essential oils that are best for cleaning include lemon, grapefruit, eucalyptus, peppermint, tea tree, lavender and rosemary.

Clove essential oil, and many others, are contained in Hildegard of Bingen's (1098-1179) medical book. She was known as the first herbalist and naturopath of the European Middle Ages. Her book documented over 12,000 remedies for various symptoms and diseases. Clove essential oil has been shown to kill dozens of strains of bacteria, fungi and a variety of viruses. Additionally, clove essential oil also was shown in research to reduce Candida by 75% after 8 days, equivalent to the use of Nystatin®, the most common pharmaceutical drug used to treat Candida.

Thieves® blend essential oil was developed based on the ingredients found in the *"Four Thieves Vinegar"* or *"Marseilles Vinegar"*, which was used to protect against the plague in the 15th Century A.D.; this essential oil blend was prepared by thieves and grave robbers who wanted protection from the plague and other ailments. Diffusing Thieves® blend of cinnamon, clove, eucalyptus, lemon and rosemary oils can kill 99% of airborne bacteria in 12

Table 6.1 Thieves® blend essential oil : properties

Cinnamon Bark (*Cinnamonum verum*) : Antiseptic, anti-viral, anti-bacterial, anti-fungal, COX inhibitor (anti-inflammatory), a strong oxygenator.

Clove (*Syzygium aromaticum*) : Antiseptic, anti-viral, anti-fungal, COX inhibitor (anti-inflammatory), one of the highest ORAC (Oxygen Radical Absorbance Capacity) values of any plant in the world!

Eucalyptus (*Eucalyptus radiata*) : Anti-inflammatory, antiseptic, anti-viral, anti-bacterial, anti-fungal, supports respiratory system.

Lemon (*Citrus limon*) : Antiseptic, immune stimulating, purifying and uplifting.

Rosemary (*Rosmarius officinalis, CT cineol*) : Antiseptic, anti-infectious, reduces mental fatigue, eases anxiety.

minutes. This makes Thieves® blend a great consideration for airline and other similar crowded travel. (Table 6.1)

How to use essential oil remedies for travel

Essential oil remedies are readily available through online Internet sources as well as numerous health stores. Through these sources, essential oils typically come as single or blended combinations in small bottles of 5-15 ml, very easy to carry on travel.

Based on the particular clinical need, as are highlighted in the sections below, one is able to choose their essential oil selection and use the drops in a diffuser or directly from the bottle to inhale, placed topically on the palmar wrists and areas of distress and rubbed in topically or taken orally as a drop or in water. It is very important to ONLY use the essential oils neat (no dilution) for those that are so indicated. Others will need to be diluted for either topical or oral use. Please also see Chapter 8 for a concise list of 12 essential oil remedies to consider for your essential oil travel first aid kit. The recommended amount of essential oil remedies should be listed on the package or container purchased, or commonly is only a drop or few drops at a time, whether used topically or internally.

Aromatic uses of essential oils on travel

When diffused into the air, essential oils can be either very stimulating for some, or calming and soothing for other oils. Beyond their emotional benefits, diffusing essential oil can even purify air of unwanted odors and some airborne pathogens. It is recommended to use diffusers with low or no-heat so as to minimize any change in the chemical structure of the oil being diffused. Rosemary, lavender, peppermint, grapefruit, chamomile, lemon and ylang-ylang essential oils have been shown to calm the mind and emotions in clinical scientific research, as well as enhancing memory recall and test performance. Clary sage helps with PMS yet should not be overused.

Topical uses of essential oils on travel

Essential oils may be easily absorbed by the skin and applied topically safely to unbroken surfaces due to their molecular micro-particle composition. Many times essential oils will have a prompt local benefit to the area treated and chamomile specifically has been shown to decrease the hives reaction. Highly favored for massage and beauty therapies, essential oils have calming as well as restorative properties and further they are natural disinfectants. Topical essential oils should usually be blended with other oils, waxes or alcohols. Citrus essential oils should not be applied when there will be direct sunlight exposure.

Essential oils that are generally regarded as safe to use undiluted on the skin include lavender, German chamomile, tea tree, sandalwood and rose geranium. It is especially important to only use half-strength oils on children and babies. For essential oils that are generally considered safe for babies and children, see Table 6.2.

Essential oils can also be used to cleanse and purify laundry and surfaces throughout the home.

Internal uses of essential oils on travel

Due to the micro-particle composition of the essential oils, they may be absorbed into the bloodstream from the skin for internal benefits. When used as dietary supplements,

Table 6.2 Essential oils generally safe for babies and children

Bergamot (*Citrus bergamia*) **
Cedarwood (*Cedrus atlantica*) **
Chamomile, Roman (*Chamaemelum nobile*)
Cypress (*Cupressus sempervirens*)
Frankincense (*Boswellia carteri*)
Geranium (*Pelargonium graveolens*)
Ginger (*Zingiber officinale*)
Lavender (*Lavandula angustifolia*)
Lemon (*Citrus limon*) **
Mandarin (*Citrus reticulata*) **
Marjoram (*Origanum majorana*)
Melaleuca (Tea Tree) (*Melaleuca alternifolia*)
Orange (*Citrus aurantium*) **
Rose Otto (*Rosa damascena*)
Rosemary (*Rosmarinus officinalis*) **
Rosewood (*Aniba rosaeodora*)
Sandalwood (*Santalum album*)
Thyme (*Thumus vulgaris, CT linalol*)
Ylang Ylang (*Cananga odorata*)

** *Always use these diluted on babies and children.*

some essential oils have been shown to have powerful anti-oxidant properties, while others help support healthy anti-inflammatory responses. While many essential oils are commonly regarded as safe for internal use, other essential oils should not be taken internally. *ONLY use essential oils internally that have the appropriate dietary supplement facts on the label.*

It is highly recommended that only 100% pure, therapeutic-grade essential oils are used in any manner, and all label warnings and instructions must be followed. CPTG®

(Certified Pure Therapeutic Grade) is the accepted standard for pure essential oils and the essential oils that carry this designation are guaranteed to be pure, natural and free of synthetic compounds or contaminates. These will be the safest and most effective essential oils available today. Essential oils should be stored in dark colored bottles and most should remain potent for 5-10 years, while citrus essential oils will retain potency for 1-2 years.

Common essential oil remedies for travel

Prevention/immunization

Use of essential oils is a very sound approach to maintaining health before and while on travel. As the oils are very concentrated, the vials or bottles of essential oils are small enough that a travel kit with several or a dozen or more will not require much space or weight in packing.

As many of the oils are known to be anti-microbial, antiseptic and immune strengthening, these should be considered by all who travel to protect from germs of many types, including bacteria, viruses and fungi. Some of the most common essential oils to consider would include lemon, grapefruit, eucalyptus, peppermint, tea tree (*Melaleuca*), lavender and rosemary. One of the greatest essential oil blends to offer protection with travel is the Thieves® blend (Figure 4.1 and text). This ancient blend has protected even grave robbers from the worst of the plague in the 15th Century A.D., as well as other travelers. Thieves® blend includes essential oils of cinnamon bark, clove, eucalyptus, lemon and rosemary.

Jet lag/ravel fatigue

Essential oils have demonstrated anti-microbial and immune support and also many are known to reinvigorate and energize people. Frankincense offers muscle relaxation and sedative support that may be very helpful to gain rest while in travel. Likewise, lemon, orange and valerian may be calming and lemongrass is said to be a revitalizer. Patchouli is reported as both a relaxant and a stimulant, as is ylang ylang. Other essential oils specifically reported as beneficial for jet lag and travel fatigue are listed in Table 6.3.

Table 6.3 Essential oils for jet lag/travel fatigue

Eucalyptus
Geranium
Grapefruit
Lavender
Peppermint

Motion sickness/sea sickness

Aiding in motion sickness will be one of the areas that will make one glad they travel with essential oils. With simply a few drops placed at the mastoid, or base of the skull behind the ears and also on the navel, relief may be quite rapid. When possible, a warm compress may be placed over the abdomen after applying the essential oil for further comfort. In addition, one may inhale the oils each 15-20 minutes as needed or even place 1-2 drops on the tongue. Essential oils to consider for motion sickness include ginger, lavender, patchouli and peppermint, among others. (Table 6.4)

Table 6.4 Essential oils for motion sickness/sea sickness

Ginger
Lavender
Patchouli
Peppermint

Cough/cold/flu

Cough, colds and flu illnesses may often be cleared with the administration of essential oils by diffusion, orally or topically. Many essential oils are anti-microbial and immune stimulants and additionally some also are mucolytic and anti-catarrhal, reducing the nasal congestion and thick mucus often accompanying these ailments.

Thieves® blend again is an all-around champion for these conditions and is both a convenient and effective blend of essential oils. Individual oils with anti-microbial benefits include blue tansy, citronella, clove, eucalyptus, frankincense, lemon, lemongrass, myrtle, patchouli, peppermint, rosemary, rosewood and tea tree essential oils. Further eucalyptus offers mucolytic and expectorant benefits, as does helichrysum, as do lemon and myrtle.

Diarrhea/dysentery/vomiting

Various essential oils calm the contractility of the gastrointestinal tract and thus may offer tremendous relief for episodes of diarrhea and vomiting. Nausea has been covered above in the section on motion sickness and in Table 6.4.

Clove is known to protect the stomach and lavender is anti-spasmodic and also a vermifuge (treats intestinal worms), as is valerian. Orange also is an anti-spasmodic and patchouli, peppermint and rosemary are digestive aids.

Essential oils should also be considered for food poisoning. Those that may prove very helpful include patchouli, peppermint, rosemary, tarragon and the Thieves[®] blend. These may be taken a few drops on the tongue or diluted in a small amount of water.

As with any other remedy for diarrhea and/or vomiting, adequate hydration remains the most critical issue and recommendations are for a person to drink 1 liter or quart for every 50 pounds or 20 kg of bodyweight daily.

Table 6.5 Essential oils for vomiting

Fennel
Lavender
Nutmeg
Patchouli
Peppermint

Pain/trauma

Trauma and pain are some of the most distressing experiences to interrupt a travel, be it for business, personal or mission purposes. Fortunately, essential oils have much to offer for pain, trauma and to aid healing.

Essential oils that have disinfectant properties may be very important for open wounds to prevent infection and to promote healing. Some of these include hyssop, oregano, tea tree, thyme and, of course, Thieves[®] blend. Helichrysum, rose otto and geranium are known to help reduce bleeding, and clove, elemi and myrrh are to be considered for infected wounds.

Essential oils that promote healing include Canadian hemlock, dorado azul, lavender and tea tree. These may be used singly or blended and applied topically 2-5 times per day, diluting as indicated per essential oil used. A great Essential Oil Natural First Aid spray is included in Table 6.6.

Table 6.6 Essential oils natural first aid spray

2 Drops Cypress
5 Drops Lavender
3 Drops Tea Tree

Blend essential oils with 1/2 teaspoon of salt.
Add blend to 8 ounces of distilled water in a spray bottle.
Shake until dissolved.

For pain while traveling, more than 60 different essential oils have been shown to have analgesic, pain relieving properties. Wintergreen essential oil contains 85-99% methyl salicylate, the same component of aspirin, thus both analgesic and anti-inflammatory in effect. Also consider peppermint as well as clove and helichrysum for muscle pains.

Dental pains can be a significant distraction on travel, and may indicate abscess or infection of the tooth root or related tissues. Essential oils that aid with relieving pains and also the infectious component include black pepper, clove, Idaho tansy, tea tree and wintergreen. With these, one may apply diluted 50:50 directly to the tooth and gum as indicated. Caution must be regarded and a competent dental professional should be consulted in the case of a possible dental infection or abscess, as serious facial and systemic sepsis infections may progress rapidly.

Table 6.7 Essential oils for insect bites

Basil
Eucalyptus
Lavender
Peppermint
Rosemary
Tea Tree

Table 6.8 Essential oils natural mosquito repellents

Basil
Blue cypress
Clove
Dorado azul
Eucalyptus globulus
Eucalyptus radiata
Geranium
Idaho Tansy
Lavender
Lemon
Lemongrass
Peppermint
Thyme

Insect bites and stings may be a real nuisance while on travel. Table 6.7 lists a number of essential oils that may be applied 1-2 drops directly on each bite or sting 3-4 times daily. In addition, Table 6.8 lists a variety of essential oils that will make great mosquito repellants, without the poisonous exposure to DEET and other toxins that are widely encouraged in the conventional medical model.

Frostbite or heat exhaustion/sunstroke

Frostbite

Essential oils may increase blood flow and provide gentle warming to frostbite tissues. Currently the recommended medical approach for frostbite is to rapidly re-warm the involved extremities, by immersing the extremities in warm water at 104-108 degrees F or 40-42 degrees C, typically for 15-30 minutes in most cases. Conventional medical care is recommended, with integrative care to further promote healing.

Some essential oils to consider include helichrysum and peppermint, as well as cypress, lavender and marjoram. Apply 1 - 2 drops of the essential oil or blend topically to the affected areas and *very gently* massage the extremities to increase circulation and to sooth the affected areas, followed by a mildly warm compress. Helichrysum is also known for nerve healing and regeneration. This approach may be repeated for a total of 2-3 treatments daily, even after the extremities are warmed, to provide relief and to promote healing.

Heat exhaustion/sunstroke

Following sunburn, lavender essential oil may be applied directly, or in a 50:50 blend to promote cooling and healing of the burned skin. Further, the lavender essential oil may be used in the manner described below, either separate or blended with the peppermint for sunstroke and heat exhaustion.

For heat exhaustion, remove clothing as is reasonably possible and apply a cool, moist washcloth to the skin, adding peppermint essential oil for cooling. The cool cloth should be drawn over the back and sides of the neck and on the palm side of the wrists for release of body heat. Peppermint essential oil increases blood flow to the skin helping your body to release heat quicker and maintain a normal body temperature. Also consider a peppermint mist in a spray bottle by adding 25 drops of peppermint essential oil in a 6-ounce water bottle and spray when you are feeling over-heated.

Contraindications of essential oils on travel

Essential oils should only be used during pregnancy under a competent physician's orders and care. Essential oils are NOT indicated for use in the eyes, the ear canal or on open wounds. One may apply any natural oil, such as extra virgin, cold pressed coconut oil or olive oil, to the affected area if redness or irritation develops while using essential oils topically.

Chapter 7
Pain Management Strategies for Travel

Safe and effective pain management on travel for business, pleasure or mission often necessitates special considerations because of remote location, extrication (evacuation) considerations and concomitant illness or injury that may impact the effects of physical modalities, pharmaceutical or natural therapeutic agents. World travelers are often exposed to various indigenous therapies for acute and chronic conditions. Many of these therapies are becoming more available to American travelers as "Complementary and Alternative Medicine" (CAM). These therapies can be integrated well with conventional medical therapies, and often may be superior to conventional approaches to the treatment of acute or chronic pain in travel settings.

The old adage, "Nobody ever died of pain", may be very inappropriate in a wilderness setting. Effective pain management may dramatically enhance a rescue effort and thus minimize morbidity and mortality. Pain management advances over the last decades have dramatically altered care in hospitals and clinics and may certainly impact care while on travel.

Physical methods for treatment of pain

Travel pain management includes simple physical measures such as applying pressure, cold, heat, or splinting, which are important adjuncts to pharmaceutical or natural therapies, and may provide significant pain relief, often with less risk.

Compression analgesia for pain on travel

Although compression is taught more as a method for establishing hemostasis (stopping bleeding) than for pain management, compression has been known to reduce pain for centuries. An injured extremity is wrapped firmly with an elastic cloth wrap (Ace® wrap) or rubber Esmarch bandage from a point on the extremity just proximal to the injury site and extending more proximally on the extremity for at least 3-4 inches and up to approximately 12 inches of compression wrapping. Alternately, a simple non-vascular occlusive constriction bandage (tourniquet) may be placed on the limb proximal to the site of the injury. Resultant pain relief is thought to occur due to compression of the peripheral nerves. Distal pulses should be evaluated and the compression wrap should allow for a palpable pulse. If the pulse is obliterated through the compression with either the wrap or tourniquet, it is essential to release the compression periodically to prevent ischemia (insufficient blood supply) in the limb. In cold environments, where the risk of ischemia is increased further, release of the compression should be more frequent to protect the tissues from ischemia. Compression analgesia may be safe and appropriate in travel settings if other therapeutic agents are unavailable or contraindicated.

Cryoanalgesia (cold therapy) for pain on travel

Hippocrates first recorded use of ice and snow packs to relieve pain in the 4th century B.C. Cryoanalgesia experienced a significant modification by Richardson in 1866 with the introduction of refrigerant ether spray, subsequently replaced by the use of ethyl chloride spray in 1890. Cooper advanced cryoanalgesia in 1961 through the development of the liquid nitrogen probe, which served as prototype for the current generation of nitrous oxide or carbon dioxide cryoanalgesia devices in common use today.

Travel cryoanalgesia may be applied with ice, snow or frigid water in adventure settings, or simply by ice or cold packs. Additionally, metal cylinders containing gasoline or ethyl alcohol remain liquid at temperatures below water's freezing point and may be used to provide a dry cold compress. These containers of sub-zero temperature liquids may lead to serious frostbite injury thus the metal container must be wrapped in cloth so as not to directly touch the skin. As cold absorbs heat from the adjacent tissues, nerve conduction is reversibly blocked. Conduction ceases in the larger myelinated fibers before the unmyelinated fibers; all nerve conduction ceases at freezing temperatures for water, $32°$ F ($0°$ C). Upon re-warming, nerve conduction resumes, unless the intracellular contents have turned to ice crystals.

While a selective cryo-lesion is the goal of many pain management treatments in chronic pain clinics, this deliberate cell injury is not appropriate in a travel setting. Prevention of frostbite and generalized hypothermia while using cold therapy is critical. The specific duration that tissue will tolerate a cold compress before experiencing cellular damage is variable, depending on pre-existent tissue hypothermia, peripheral versus central nature of the tissue, and temperature and pressure of the cold compress. Cold-water immersion may induce frostbite in persons with snakebite due to venom-compromised tissues. Cold packs are shown to be beneficial for certain marine envenomations. Commercial cold packs typically contain a gel of water and propylene glycol, or other similar antifreeze and heat exchange substances, which may be cooled in cold water or snow. A reasonable guide is to place a dry thin cotton cloth or foam between the skin and cold metal cylinders, ice, snow or cold packs and to remove cold therapy each 15 minutes to assess tissue status.

Heat therapy for pain on travel

Application of heat is not usually recommended for initial (up to 48 hours) pain management of acute trauma, because it may lead to increased edema and bleeding. There are, however, reasonable applications for the use of heat for pain management in travel. Muscle relaxation, attributed to decreased gamma fiber activity, has been demonstrated after applying heat to the overlying skin. Collagen tissues become more extensible with heat therapy, requiring less force for movement and resulting in less mechanical damage with stretching. These effects may be useful for patients pursuing wilderness travel, especially with chronic pain conditions. Further, heat applied to the skin of the abdomen may markedly reduce gastrointestinal peristalsis and uterine contractions and thus decrease pain associated with these organs.

Application of heat need not be extreme. Temperatures in the range of 100 to 104° F (37.8 to 40° C) for 10 to 20 minutes will generally be comforting, without leading to thermal injury. Heat therapy should be avoided in patients who are cognitively impaired and should be avoided on tissue that is anesthetic or ischemic, to prevent further unintended tissue injury. Heat therapy may worsen marine envenomations or lead to lymphangitis.

Liniments and balms are not true heat transfer agents; rather, they typically consist of multiple botanical or chemical substances that make the tissue feel warm through counter-irritant effects and subsequent vasodilation. Through this vasodilatation, these substances may help a traveler's pain and stiffness abate. Common ingredients include menthol, camphor, mustard oil, eucalyptus oil, methyl nicotinate, methyl salicylate and wormwood oil. These products are generally only recommended on intact skin with a light cloth or plastic covering and should not be placed on mucous membranes. They also should not be used with tight compresses or external heat sources.

Splinting for pain and trauma on travel

Splinting allows positioning and immobilization of injured body parts and prevents further damage to soft tissues, blood vessels, nerves, and bones. Preventing bony fragments from damaging surrounding tissue diminishes pain and often facilitates mobilization and extrication of a victim. Splinting should be applied at a minimum of one bony segment proximal and one bony segment below distal to the injury in question for stabilization.

Splints should be padded to prevent further surface trauma. They may be accompanied by pressure dressings or cold compresses for additional pain management. Regular re-evaluation of tissue circulatory status is critical to prevent damage from swelling, frostbite or ischemia in immobile, splinted limbs. Splinting should not inadvertently act as a tourniquet to obstruct blood flow, unless that is necessary for the nature of the specific injury. If tourniquet placement is important, periodic loosening should be considered if there is no limb amputated beyond the tourniquet. When loosening a tourniquet, be sure to do so slowly and keep the tourniquet otherwise in place so it may be tightened once again if there is significant blood loss. Recommendations in medical literature are highly variable; if extrication and emergency professional care is more than 2-4 hours beyond placement of the tourniquet, periodic loosening should be considered carefully each 1-2 hours. Rapid consultation with competent healthcare emergency professionals is recommended always for serious trauma.

Magnet therapy

Magnetic therapy has been described for approximately 4000 years in the Hindu *Vedas* and in the Chinese acupuncture classic, *Huang Te Nei Ching.* The application of magnetic stones, or "lodestones", is said in ancient legends of Cleopatra and others to have decreased pain and preserved youth. Early Romans used the discharge of the electric eel to treat arthritis and gout, perhaps the earliest known electro-magnetic therapy.

Danish physicist Oerstad proved in 1820 that an electric current flowing through a wire had its own magnetic field. Modern medicine's most familiar use of magnetic energy is with Magnetic Resonance Imaging (MRI) imaging. There are various theories about the effectiveness of permanent magnets for use in pain and healing. Some researchers have reported increased blood circulation and increased macrophage activity, and others have hypothesized effects on peripheral nerves, including blockage or modification of sensory neuron action potentials and enhanced regeneration of peripheral nerves.

Most permanent magnets marketed at this time for management of pain measure approximately 200 to 1200 gauss in strength. At this level, there is little, if any, risk in trying a magnet for pain reduction, as this author has seen benefits personally and in his pain medicine practice with magnets over many years. Many patients report significant pain reduction within minutes to hours, while others report relief after wearing the magnets for several days or more. In business, personal and mission travel, it is reasonable to carry a few therapeutic magnets, as they are usually lightweight, compact and unbreakable. It is very important to pack these therapeutic magnets away from electronics as they may damage these with their magnetic force.

Magnets marketed for pain therapy range in size from a 2-inch circle to a 6 x 12 inch rectangular pad. Most are only a few millimeters thick and are often flexible. These are becoming more readily available through multi-level marketing, television "infomercials," health food stores and the Internet. Some people have also experienced pain relief with simple, small magnets such as those used to place notes and photographs on a refrigerator. Generally, placement of the magnet should be directly over the area of pain, and it should be held in place with tape, clothing, or straps.

A premier approach to magnetic therapy is through the remarkable work of Robert D. Milne, M.D. His Micro-Vibrational Therapy (MVT) Personal Relief Assistant (PRA) is a remarkable tool for pain management. The MVT is compact, handheld and highly effective for numerous pain conditions, balancing the body through micro-vibrational, magnetic, sonar and LED light energies to promote pain relief and healing (see Resources).

Botanical/herbal remedies for pain on travel

The term "herb" is broadly defined as a non-woody plant that dies down to the ground after flowering. The term "botanical" is a more general description of flora, although common interpretation describes any plant used for medicinal therapy, nutritional value or food seasoning or dyeing (coloring). As with acupuncture, homeopathy and other natural therapeutics, the use of botanicals may be encountered in travel settings as a part of the indigenous culture and medical care. Botanicals are often prepared as teas or infusions, with the plant's soft portions placed in a pot and covered by boiling water to create a supernatant. Herbal decoctions are traditionally prepared in special earthen crocks, or in containers of stainless steel, ceramic, or enamel by contemporary practitioners, specifically avoiding aluminum and alloy metal pots. The herb is placed in the container and covered with cold water that is then boiled, covered and simmered.

Travelers may encounter an herbal remedy dispensed as a poultice, botanical liniment, ointment or oil to be applied to the skin. Alternately, many modern herbalists utilize capsule forms of herbs for ease of administration. Combinations of several herbs are often more effective than a single herb, and common formulae have been recorded worldwide for centuries. Appropriate application or prescription of botanical products rarely leads to toxicity or adverse reactions, although such are possible if botanicals are used excessively or carelessly.

Certain botanical products that have been used for pain include morphine, isolated from the opium poppy (*Papaver somniferum*) and cocaine, from Coca leaves (*Erythroxylum coca*). Often used as a seasoning or food, oregano (*Oreganum vulgare*) has been reported to be beneficial for rheumatic pain. Sunflower (*Helianthus annuus*) is a source of phenylalanine, useful for general pain. Turmeric (*Curcuma longa*) contains curcumin, an anti-inflammatory substance which is beneficial for rheumatoid arthritis, and ginger (*Zingiber officinale*) is beneficial for rheumatoid arthritis, osteoarthritis and fibromyalgia. Clove (*Syzygium aromaticum*) is endorsed by the German botanical resource Commission E topically for dental pain. Red peppers (*Capsicum species*) contain Substance P-depleting capsaicin and also salicylates (aspirin-type compounds). Often taken as an infusion or decoction, kava kava (*Piper methysticum*) contains both dihydrokavain and dihydromethysticin, which have analgesic effectiveness similar to that of aspirin, and evening primrose (*Oenothera biennis*) is a great source of tryptophan and has been demonstrated to relieve pain associated with diabetic neuropathy. Lavender (*Lavandula* species) contains linalool and linalyl aldehyde, which appear to be useful for pain of burns and other injuries in topical and aromatherapy form.

Willow (*Salix* species), which has been used to treat pain since 500 B.C., contains salicin and other salicylate (aspirin-type) compounds. Commission E has recognized willow as an effective pain reliever for headaches, arthritis, and many other pains.

Other salicylate containing plants include red peppers, wintergreen, and birch bark. *All botanicals containing salicylates should be avoided in persons who are sensitive or allergic to aspirin products. Further, children who have viral infections such as a cold or influenza should avoid these products, as salicylates have been implicated in the development of Reye's syndrome.*

Chamomile (*Matricaria chamomilla*) contains chamazulene, which is reportedly beneficial for abdominal pain related to gastrointestinal spasm or colic; as an antihistaminic, it has mild calming or sedative properties. It is used in Europe to treat leg ulcers and may be beneficial for painful, irritated bites and stings. Plantain major (*Plantago major*) is also commonly useful for bites and stings, poison ivy discomfort, and toothache, and has been used traditionally by Native Americans as a wound dressing. Aloe gel (*Aloe vera*) has been used since ancient times to treat burns and sunburn and to promote wound healing.

Especially useful for sprains and strains is the mountain daisy or Arnica (*Arnica montana*), which is also endorsed by the German Commission E. Arnica was in the U.S. Pharmacopoeia in the early 1800s to 1960s and has long been used by Native Americans and others for relieving back pain and other myofascial pains and bruising. It is used topically or internally, often in homeopathic form. Comfrey (*Symphytum officinale*) has been used since ancient Greece for skin problems. It contains alloin, which is anti-inflammatory, and is endorsed by Commission E to topically treat bruises, dislocations, and sprains. Comfrey has experienced a controversial safety record because oral

Table 7.1 Botanical/herbal remedies for pain on travel : indications

Aloe gel : burns, sunburn
Arnica Montana : sprains, strains, bruises, injuries
Birch bark : aspirin-like pain effect, general pain relief
Chamomile : abdominal pain, spasm or colic, leg ulcers, bites, stings
Clove : dental pain
Coca leaves : morphine-like effect, general pain relief
Comfrey : skin problems
Curcumin : general pain effects, potent anti-inflammatory
Evening primrose : diabetic neuropathy
Ginger : arthritis, fibromyalgia, Rheumatic pains
Kava kava : aspirin-like pain effect, general pain relief
Lavender : burns, abrasions
Oregano : Rheumatic pains
Plantain major : bites, stings, poison ivy, toothache, wound dressing
Red peppers : aspirin-like pain effect, general pain relief
Sunflower : general pain relief
Willow : aspirin-like pain effect, headache, arthritis
Wintergreen : aspirin-like pain effect

ingestion of its pyrrolizidine alkaloids has been associated with hepato-toxicity and/or carcinogenicity. For this reason, only topical use of comfrey is recommended.

Finally, as with pharmaceutical medical care, adjuvant medications may add pain relief to those botanical agents selected which further are indicated for anxiety and depression. In fact, utilizing both remedies together often requires less of each botanical or pharmaceutical remedy than if using either separately.

Botanical considerations for anxiety and depression include licorice, with its eight licorice compounds exhibiting MAOI (Mono-Amine Oxidase Inhibitor) effects, which are also seen in many pharmaceutical preparations. An easy way to use licorice is to add it into teas. Use should be moderate to about 1-3 cups daily, as excess use may produce hypertension, headaches and lethargy. Siberian ginseng (*Eleutherococcus senticosus*) also acts as an MAO Inhibitor and often improves a sense of wellbeing. This is available either in capsules or as an extract.

St. John's Wort (see Chapter 4, Botanical/Herbal Remedies for Travel) has a long folk history of use for anxiety and depression, often with very pleasing results. Some studies have even shown its active ingredient, hypericin, to be more effective than pharmaceutical drugs like amitriptyline (Elavil®) and imipramine (Tofranil®), and with fewer side effects, if any. Further, St. John's Wort has shown enhanced sleep quality, often a problem for those in pain.

Ginger (*Zingiber officinale*) not only has uplifting flavor, it also uplifts mood and is often effective for anxiety and depression. It also has a long folk history of efficacy.

Purslane (*Portulaca oleracea*) is rich in magnesium and potassium, which are shown to have anti-depressant properties as well as also containing calcium, folate and lithium. Purslane contains up to 16% anti-depressant compounds on a dry weight basis.

Thyme (*Thymus vulgaris*) is rich in the anti-depressant mineral lithium and gingko (*Gingko biloba*) has demonstrated improvement in brain blood flow and improved mood with 80 mg. of gingko extract three times daily in patients who were unresponsive to pharmaceutical anti-depressants.

Vitamin B-rich foods should also be considered to improve mood and allay anxiety. These help to keep neurotransmitter levels high which are essential for nerve cells to communicate and function properly. Good sources of folate include asparagus, broccoli, Brussels sprouts, navy beans, okra, pinto beans and spinach. Vitamin B6 (pyridoxine) is present in high levels in bananas, broccoli, Brussels sprouts, cauliflower, kale, peas, radishes and squash.

Table 7.2 Botanical/herbal remedies for adjuvant pain therapy on travel

B Vitamin foods
Ginger
Gingko
Licorice
Purslane
Siberian ginseng
St. John's Wort
Thyme

Homeopathic remedies for pain on travel

Homeopathic remedies have long been effective for many with pain and should be very useful for travel. As with botanical/herbal remedies, the risk of side effects is minimal and potential benefit is often profound. The following information is also found in Chapter 5, Homeopathic Remedies for Travel, along with a more comprehensive discussion of homeopathy.

Arnica Montana is likely the most widely recognized remedy for relieving pain from trauma. A North American native flower, the Mountain Daisy or Coneflower, this plant is often used in gross botanical preparations and also in homeopathic remedies. Some authors consider it useful in prophylactic considerations as well as symptomatically.

Table 7.3 Homeopathic remedies for pain/trauma : indications

Arnica Montana : general pain remedy, swelling, prophylactic use

Aconitum napellus : eye injuries ("Arnica of the eye"), shock and great fear, natural disasters, accidents

Apis mellifica : swelling, burning, stinging pain

Arsenicum album : burns, especially 1st and 2nd degree

Bellis perennis : Bruises, arthritis

Bryonia alba : Cough, sprains worse with motion, mastitis (breast inflammation), fractured ribs

Calendula : abrasions, incised wounds

Cantharis : Burns, especially 2nd and 3rd degree, urinary tract infections

Euptorium : fractures of bones

Hypericum perfollatum : Sharp and shooting pains, especially nerve, compound fractures, corneal eye injuries, dental pain, injury to nerves, to coccyx

Staphysagria is another common homeopathic remedy for pain and trauma. Specifically it is recommended for trauma that is particularly intrusive to a person, where there is a strong sense of personal violation.

Other homeopathic pain/trauma remedies with their specific associations are included in Table 7.3.

Table 7.3 Homeopathic remedies for pain/trauma : indications, (continued)

Ledum palustre : penetrating injuries, bites and stings, splinters, black eye
Natrum sulphuricum : head injury
Rhus toxicodendron : sprains and strains, especially when worse in cold, damp weather
Ruta graveolans : tendon strains, Carpal Tunnel Syndrome, eyestrain
Staphysagria : incised wounds, urethral dilation
Symphytum : fractures of bones, eye pain
Urtical urens : stings, hives, burning and itching symptoms

Essential oil remedies for pain on travel

While Chapter 6 describes the use of essential oils for a broad range of opportunities to maintain or regain health while on travel, essential oils for use in pain management are important not only for decreasing the experience of pain, yet also for promoting healing of injured tissue, regeneration of nerves, relaxation of frayed emotions and to soothe one recovering from accident, illness or injury that is associated with pain.

As noted before, many essential oils have demonstrated analgesic or pain relieving properties. Wintergreen essential oil contains 85-99% methyl salicylate, the same component of aspirin, thus both analgesic and anti-inflammatory in effect. Also consider peppermint as well as clove and helichrysum for muscle pains. (Table 7.4) These separate or blended oils may be massaged in a 50:50 dilution into sore muscles 3-4 times daily.

Table 7.4 Essential oils for muscle pain

Clove
Helichrysum
Peppermint
Wintergreen

Joint pains may often respond to topical, oral or inhaled essential oils of balsam fir, Douglas fir, nutmeg, peppermint, Roman chamomile, spruce and wintergreen. Essential oils effect not only pain relief; they may also promote healing. (Table 7.5) Consider massaging the affected joints with a 50:50 dilution of the single or blended essential oils 3-4 times daily.

Table 7.5 Essential oils for joint pain

Balsam Fir
Douglas Fir
Nutmeg
Peppermint
Roman Chamomile
Spruce
Wintergreen

Some travelers experience pain on a daily or nearly daily basis for months or years due to a variety of conditions. Essential oils that have demonstrated benefit for chronic pain include balsam fir, basil, clove, Douglas fir, helichrysum, Idaho tansy, peppermint, valerian and wintergreen (Table 7.6). Depending on the location of the chronic pain, commonly the area involved may be rubbed with a 50:50 dilution of single or blended essential oils 3-4 times daily. Additionally, chronic pain sufferers will commonly be aided with inhalation of diffusion or with a couple of drops of the essential oil on the tongue.

Table 7.6 Essential oils for chronic pain

Balsam Fir
Basil
Clove
Douglas Fir
Helichrysum
Idaho Tansy
Peppermint
Valerian
Wintergreen

Dental pain

Essential oils that aid with relieving pains and also the infectious component of dental problems include black pepper, clove, Idaho tansy, tea tree and wintergreen. One may apply diluted 50:50 directly to the tooth and gum as indicated. Caution must be regarded and a competent dental professional should be consulted in the case of a possible dental infection or abscess, as serious facial and systemic sepsis infections may progress rapidly!

Acupuncture for pain management on travel

Acupuncture developed over the last 3 to 5 millennia in Asia, and has also been practiced over the past several hundred years in the western world. Even in the USA, acupuncture has been practiced by physicians for approximately 200 years, as is documented in medical literature.

In many cases, acupuncture developed in geographic and social conditions very similar to the primitive or undeveloped conditions familiar to travelers, especially in adventure travel settings. The use of acupuncture by physicians to treat trauma and illness in wilderness settings has been described recently in medical literature. Properly administered acupuncture should have a very low risk of morbidity and may be extremely effective in alleviating pain and even restoring function to an injured traveler. Many parts of the world now have acupuncture practitioners who may be consulted for travel pain and other issues.

As there is much confusion in the American public about acupuncture and practitioners, a brief consideration is worthwhile. Contemporary medical acupuncturists are typically trained in a variety of styles or traditions, although in the USA, many physician acupuncturists and most non-physician acupuncturists have a heavy influence of only the Traditional Chinese Medicine (TCM) acupuncture paradigm. A combined approach of acupuncture point selections based on neuro-anatomy and those that are felt to have energetic effects in the body is this author's preference. Most Chiropractors study and become certified in acupuncture, especially anatomical acupuncture, through their professional organizations. Additionally, acupuncture micro-systems are often employed, where the entire body is represented in a small area such as the ear, scalp, or hand. These micro-systems are often quite beneficial for acute and/or chronic pain.

Case examples of acupuncture treatment for pain on travel

The following cases are presented to acquaint the reader with a range of experiences the author has had with using acupuncture while in travel settings, often wilderness, adventure travel or in mission travel settings. While the details will be more technical than most lay readers will understand, hopefully the cases will demonstrate the usefulness of acupuncture and have one consider acupuncture care while on travel.

A common clinical case that often responds to acupuncture is a sprained ankle. An energetic style of acupuncture that is especially useful for common trauma utilizes the Tendino-Muscular Meridians (TMM) of the acupuncture energetic subsystems. The indications for activation of the TMM treatment include acute strains, sprains, abrasions, and hematomas. The method of activation for this style of treatment is to place a needle in the *Jing-well* point (Opening Point) of one to three of the meridians involved in the lesion. This is followed by placing a needle in the "Gathering Point" for the meridian(s), then by placement of needles approximately 1 cm around the area of induration, swelling, or bruising (Figure 7.1). All needles in this treatment are place to only 1 to 3 mm depth and are left in place for 20 to 45 minutes.

Commonly, a lateral ankle sprain involves both the Gall Bladder and Bladder TMM zones. The *Jing-well* Points for these meridians are at GB 44 and BL 67 on the lateral angles of the 4th and 5th toes, respectively. The Gathering Point for these meridians is at SI 18, just below the zygoma (cheek bone) in line with the lateral canthus (outer border of the eye). Local needles typically include 4 to 6 placed around the swelling or ecchymosis (bruising) of the ankle sprain. Recovery from the sprain may proceed much more rapidly with this type of acupuncture input than with conventional therapies of rest-ice-compression-elevation (R-I-C-E) alone. Failure to respond with 70 to 85% or greater decrease in pain over 24 to 48 hours may, in fact, alert the medical acupuncturist that an injury may be more serious than initially appreciated.

Figure 7.1 TMM acupuncture treatment for ankle sprain

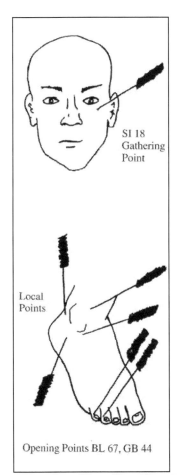

SI 18
Gathering
Point

Local
Points

Opening Points BL 67, GB 44

Most acupuncture treatments will require substantial training to be responsibly integrated with conventional western therapies. National and international standards of training have been established for western-trained physicians who desire to incorporate acupuncture into their traditional medical practices. The American Academy of Medical Acupuncture (AAMA) is the professional organization representing U.S. physician acupuncturists whose training meets or exceeds standards established by the World Health Organization's affiliate, the World Federation of Acupuncture and Moxibustion Societies. The National Commission for Certification of Acupuncture and Oriental Medicine provides testing and resources primarily for U.S.

non-physician acupuncturists. The International Council of Medical Acupuncture and Related Techniques (ICMART) is comprised of approximately 90 physician acupuncture organizations representing more than 30,000 medical acupuncturists from around the world and provides international educational congresses and symposia.

Auricular Therapy for pain on travel

Acupuncture micro-systems have been a part of sophisticated health care for thousands of years, perhaps (likely) predating even the comprehensive organization of body acupuncture. Ancient Egyptian illustrations showing treatments of the whole body through stimulating specific parts of the body, including foot therapy, hand therapy, and auricular (ear) therapy, may represent the oldest practices that have emerged to be recognized as the acupuncture *micro-systems*. Other micro-systems with ancient origins include the reflex diagnostic systems of the Chinese radial artery pulses and the tongue and abdominal diagnosis such as with Japanese Hara Diagnosis, among others. Advanced micro-systems have developed with great sophistication in the last forty years in the areas of the scalp, hands, and the ears. While the ancients were known to treat the body's physiological and pain problems with points in each of these areas, no truly sophisticated system of organization was developed until contemporary times, particularly for the hand, the scalp and the ear.

More contemporary or "conventional" medicine has also recognized the micro-system organizations. Head's Zones, described by noted British Sir Henry Head, are skin surface or cutaneous (skin surface) projections of organ or deep structure pathologies as they project their information to the body surface. Cutaneo-visceral and viscero-cutaneous reflexes are recognized to be projections of information from the skin to the organs or the organs to the skin, respectively.

Korean Dr. Tae Woo Yoo and others have developed highly sophisticated micro-systems of the hand, wherein the entire body may be treated at various levels of complexity, with stimulation only on the hands. In fact, some acupuncturists work within various traditions or paradigms of acupuncture and yet only stimulate the hand points of this micro-system and report clinical response as effective as those seen with similar treatments using body acupuncture stimulation. This author has expanded or modified the hand therapy charts to include newer findings for advanced pathologies (Figures 7.2 and 7.3 and Resources).

Figure 7.2 Hand Therapy reflex charts

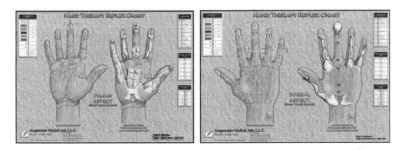

Figure 7.3 Hand Therapy advanced phases charts

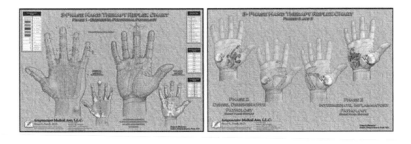

Auricular Therapy or auriculotherapy has emerged as the leading acupuncture micro-system around the world since the 1950s. Perhaps the earliest use of the ear comes from the Egyptians, who pierced the lobule (lobe) of the ear to stimulate visual clarity for their seafaring endeavors. Hippocrates mentions auricular stimulation for impotence in the 4th century B.C. As noted above, the Chinese certainly used various ear points in their acupuncture models for treatment, though not as a part of a complex organization as later evolved. Various physicians in Europe in the 1600s through the 1800s wrote of auricular (ear) stimulation in the medical literature of their day, usually for treatment of back pain or sciatica (referred pain down the leg from sciatic nerve symptoms from pathology in the lower back), and also for dental pain and other ailments. Even Dr. Rulker of Cincinnati, Ohio wrote of auricular stimulation for the treatment of sciatica in American medical literature.

For contemporary practitioners, Auricular Therapy is clearly organized and may be learned in a relatively short period of time, and even lay users may become quite adept. Many physicians, chiropractors, dentists, acupuncturists, detoxification technicians and other therapists now practice Auricular Therapy. Texts, atlases, and charts of the body's projections to the ear have become increasingly available, especially over the last several decades. This author began to use the term "Auricular Therapy" in the mid-1990s rather than the earlier term auriculotherapy in order to more clearly distinguish his presentations from other more simplified presentations commonly seen and taught today.

Auricular Therapy is the predominant acupuncture micro-system, and it is remarkably applicable for travel. Many times a lay person may effectively use the maps that indicate the points on the ear that correspond to body parts that may be experiencing pain. With simple stimulation of these identified points, pain is minimized or eliminated within minutes or after periodic repeated treatments.

"The Man in the Ear"

The Father of Auricular Therapy is rightly recognized internationally as the French physician, Dr. Paul Nogier. From the early 1950s until his death in 1996, Dr. Nogier led an international group of physicians in remarkable discoveries of the ear as a diagnostic and treatment opportunity. Dr. Nogier discovered a truly remarkable and sophisticated projection of the body to the ear. All organs, structures, and tissues have been identified in their locations on the ear, and recent studies using f-MRI imaging is demonstrating what he and his colleagues showed clinically many years before.

For instance, recent studies by Alimi show that if the right thumb is clamped, certain specific areas of the brain will become activated and these areas are detectable on the imaging scans of the brain. Similarly, when the right thumb point as projected to the ear is stimulated, areas of the brain that are activated are nearly identical to those shown with clamping onto the thumb itself. While still early, concerted research may unveil many of the mysteries of the auricular model over the next decades.

Beyond the vertebral column or spine that was initially discovered, Dr. Nogier went on to identify 30 key anatomical points in his earliest illustrations, and these subsequently revealed a projection of the human form in an inverted or upside-down position, such as a fetus in the womb (see Figure 7.4). Thus, the term "inverted fetus" is commonly used to describe the overall projection of the body to the ear. While the casual illustrations of this inverted fetus show the projection in general terms, the actual projections are very specific (Figure 7.5 and Resources). For example, one may find very specific zones for the projection of the shoulder, the knee, the liver, gall bladder, various brain structures, or of virtually any structure, whether it is musculo-skeletal, organ, or brain structure onto the ear.

Figure 7.4 "Inverted fetus"

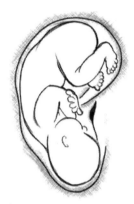

With basic exam using a probe, an electrical detection device (as is used by most professional Auricular Therapy practitioners) or simply with one's own fingernail, an active or tender point may be identified with the aid of the available auricular maps and one will often find correlation between the body pain or dysfunction and the point or points on the ear. Then, with simple gentle stimulation by an acupuncture needle, a micro-current electrical device (as is used by most professional Auricular Therapy practitioners), or again, simply one's fingernail, the

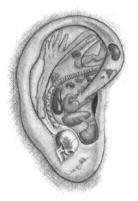

stimulus will be sent to the brain and then to the body part in question. Many times while on adventure travel such as trekking or backpacking, this author has utilized this simple fingernail method of finding and treating active, tender auricular points with great success.

Figure 7.5 Phase I auricular projections

Beyond this simple "inverted fetus" (Phase 1) presentation presented above, Dr. Nogier and his colleagues went on to further identify Phases 2 and 3, which represent dense, degenerative pathology and also intermediate, inflammatory pathology, respectively. These Phases are presented with great precision in available charts and if there is not success using the simple Phase 1 presentation, the others should be considered as well. A good presentation of Auricular Therapy for laymen is presented in the author's book, *Layman's Guide to Auricular Therapy: Amazing medicine-free healing of pain, addictions and medical problems through Auricular Therapy* (see Resources).

Table 7.7 Simplified instructions for Auricular Therapy reference chart

A comprehensive seminar is strongly recommended for Auricular Therapy practitioners to fully understand the development and importance of approaching the patient and their conditions in a full Phase approach. While not all patients respond even to advanced Auricular Therapy, many more will do so when conditions are approached using the 3-Phase model. This chart may also be useful for patients' self-care between clinic visits (see Figures 7.1, 7.2, 7.3, 7.4, 7.5 and Resources).

To assist new and seasoned therapists and also patients in the use of this Reference Card, please consider the following:
1. All clinical conditions *may* exist in one, two, or three Phase presentations concurrently, depending on the patho-physiology of the condition.
2. When searching for the auricular projection(s) of the various anatomical tissues or structures, examine the ear for the projection(s) of a given

structure in each of the three Phases, using a probe, electrical detector or one's fingernail. For example, if the shoulder is hurting, scan for its location in each of the 3-Phase locations as presented on the Reference Card.

3. If one or more of the Phase projections of the tissue is active (electrically detectable with a point finder or manually detectable and tender to probing), you may treat the active point(s).

4. If the point(s) are not active or detectable with your point finder, they do not need to be treated.

5. Always consider the possible etiology or cause of a condition, rather than just treating symptoms. For example, if a condition of the forearm is not responding to treatment even in the 3-Phase approach, consider scanning for the 3 Phases of the cervical spine, spinal cord or cervical spinal nerves.

6. We recommend setting the detection sensitivity of the electrical stimulators with a general scan of the ear prior to actual auricular examination. Set the sensitivity of the device where a general scan of the upper, middle and lower ear gives only one or two positive signals. Then, scan in specific locations according to the auricular maps. If many points are active on the initial general scan, decrease the sensitivity and re-scan to a setting where only one or two points are active on the general pre-scanning.

7. Many times the treatment will be more effective by treating a few points with proper selection, rather than many points with a casual or haphazard approach.

The zonal presentations found in the *Pocket Atlas of Auricular Therapy and Auricular Medicine* and the text,

Auricular Medicine and Auricular Therapy: A Practical Approach, are highly recommended to complement the anatomical presentations of the Desk Reference Card (see References).

Chapter 8
Natural First Aid Kits for Travel

With the knowledge gained from this writing regarding a variety of natural or integrative therapeutics for the traveler to stay well or get well while on travel, travelers should always prepare and carry basic supplies in a personal travel wellness first aid kit. This is important both for domestic travel and is especially important for international travel, as familiar resources and professional help may not be readily accessible.

It is not expected that one would take *all* the possible remedies that are presented in this book. Based on the familiarity of various remedies and those which are learned in this writing, generally one should start with Structured Silver and activated charcoal and then either a botanical, homeopathic or essential oil set of remedies.

Structured Silver and activated charcoal should be in EVERY travel first aid kit! The broad indications coupled with remarkable safety make Structured Silver and activated charcoal two of the most effective and yet safest natural remedies for a wide variety of clinical conditions.

Table 8.1 Essential first aid travel kit, ALWAYS carry

Structured Silver: liquid, gel
Activated charcoal: powder, capsules, tablets, salve

GMP always travels with both liquid and gel forms of Structured Silver as well as powder and capsules of activated charcoal. Structured Silver is used on a preventative basis daily during the week before, during and for the week following international travel. If illness threatens, dosing of the Structured Silver and the activated charcoal may be increased as indicated. Resources for obtaining these as well as botanical, homeopathic and essential oil remedies are included in the Resources section of this book.

Tables 8.1, 8.2, 8.3 and 8.4 give concise recommendations of travel first aid kits including foremost Structured Silver and activated charcoal, and then within the botanical, homeopathic and essential oil remedy lines. In each, only twelve remedies have been proposed, as not to overwhelm the traveler with too many remedies either by cost or bulk. As one begins with these basics and then learns through reading and research and personal experience, the first aid kit may be modified to the particular needs of those traveling and to the specific destinations. Again, *always consult with a competent healthcare professional in the event of illness while on travel.*

How to use botanical/herbal remedies for travel

Botanical and herbal remedies are readily available through online Internet sources as well as numerous health stores. Through these sources, botanicals are commonly in dried, loose-leaf form to make teas and poultices, as tinctures and commonly as single or combination products in capsules. Many will find the tinctures and capsules to be the easiest to carry on travel.

Based on the particular clinical need, as are highlighted in the sections below, one is able to choose their botanical selection and then take orally as a tea, tincture or capsule or topically as a poultice. The recommended amount of botanical/herbal products should be listed on the package or container purchased.

Table 8.2 Botanical/herbal first aid kit, 12 remedies :
indications

Aloe vera gel, liquid, powder capsules : promotes healing,
burns, sunburn, abrasions, cuts, hives, frostbite,
gastrointestinal distress, constipation

Anise : mucolytic, expectorant, anti-viral

Arnica ointment, capsules, tea, tincture : disinfecting,
wound healing, sprains, strains, bruises,
dislocations, muscle pain, joint pain, bites, stings,
sunburn

Calendula gel, ointment, tincture : cuts, bruises, anti-
inflammatory, bites, stings, sunburn, anti-bacterial,
anti-viral, anti-fungal

Chamomile tincture : relaxant, somnolent, anti-bacterial,
anti-viral, immune support, stings

Echinacea tincture or capsules : immune support, cough,
colds, flu, anti-bacterial, anti viral,   anti-fungal,
wound repair

Gingko biloba extracts, tinctures, capsules: enhanced
circulation, arrhythmias, altitude sickness,
hangover, headache, frostbite, anti-oxidant, free
radical scavenger, immune support

Hypericum (St. John's Wort) capsule, ointment, tincture,
tea : jet lag, sedative, anxiolytic, antidepressant,
bites, stings, scabies, bruises, cuts, burns, sunburn
avoid in pregnancy and caution with sunlight

Plantago capsule, tincture, tea : diarrhea, constipation,
burns, sunburn, bites, stings, poison ivy, laryngitis,
pharyngitis, anti-bacterial, astringent

Valerian capsules, tincture, tea : jet lag, sedative, anti-
anxiety, arrhythmias, palpitations, improves
circulation, lowers high blood pressure, improves
cardiac output, gastrointestinal spasm

Table 8.2 Botanical/herbal first aid kit, 12 remedies : indications, continued

Compound botanical remedies:

Coix Formula® : motion sickness, food poisoning, excessive eating and drinking alcohol, nausea, headache, vomiting, diarrhea or constipation, gastrointestinal cramping, generalized pain.

Zheng Gu Shui : sprains, strains, bruises, muscle pain, arthritis pain.

How to use homeopathic remedies for travel

Homeopathic remedies are readily available through online Internet sources as well as numerous health stores. Through these sources, homeopathic remedies are commonly available for oral use as small pellets or as liquid drops or spays commonly used sublingually (under the tongue) and topically as creams or gels. All of these forms are easy to carry on travel.

Based on the particular clinical need, as are highlighted in the sections below, one is able to choose their homeopathic remedy selection and then take orally as pellets, drops or spray under the tongue or topically as a cream or gel. The recommended amount of homeopathic remedies may be listed on the package or container purchased.

Unless otherwise noted, for acute injuries and illnesses, most homeopathic preparations should be considered in 3X, 6X or 12X potency and given every 15-30 minutes immediately after injury or onset until symptoms improve. Typically 2-3 pellets or 2-3 drops of homeopathic liquid under the tongue are adequate. If no effect is noticed after 2-3 doses, the homeopathic selection should be reconsidered. Aconite 3X plus Bryonia 3X may be a trusted

Table 8.3 Homeopathic first aid kit, 12 remedies : indications

Arnica Montana : general pain remedy, swelling, bruising, trauma, overexertion, prophylactic use

Aconitum napellus : eye injuries ("Arnica of the eye"), shock and great fear, natural disasters, accidents

Apis mellifica : swelling, burning, stinging pain, hives, anaphylaxis

Arsenicum album : gastroenteritis, food poisoning, burns, especially 1st and 2nd degree

Belladona : headaches, seizures, vertigo, pharyngitis, bronchitis, tonsillitis, sinusitis, epistaxis (nosebleed), inflammations, constipation, cystitis, influenza

Coccolus indica : motion sickness, jet lag, restore sleep cycle

Hypericum perfollatum : Sharp and shooting pains, especially nerve, compound fractures, corneal eye injuries, snake bites, dental pain, injury to nerves and to coccyx, 1st and 2nd degree burns

Ledum palustre : penetrating injuries, bites and stings, splinters, black eye

Nux vomica : nausea, heartburn, headache, hangover, vertigo, gastrointestinal cramping, colic, cystitis, allergic rhinitis, cough, asthma, sinusitis, pain, stiffness

Ossilicoccinum : influenza, headaches, body aches, fever, chills, fatigue, H1N1 swine flu

Rhus toxicodendron : sprains and strains, especially when worse in cold, damp weather, poison ivy, oak or sumac, general connective tissue swelling, arthritis, bronchitis, overexertion, shingles, hives, angina

Complex homeopathic remedy:

Traumeel® : sprains, strains, contusions, bruises, pain,

Table 8.3 Homeopathic first aid kit, 12 remedies : indications

first aid remedy for nearly all acute illnesses, taking 5-10 drops under the tongue every 15 minutes for 2-3 hours, as needed.

How to use essential oil remedies for travel

Essential oil remedies are readily available through online Internet sources as well as numerous health stores. Through these sources, essential oils typically come as single or blended combinations in small bottles of 5-15 ml, very easy to carry on travel.

Based on the particular clinical need, as are highlighted in the sections below, one is able to choose their essential oil selection and use the drops in a diffuser or directly from the bottle to inhale, placed topically on the palmar wrists and areas of distress and rubbed in topically or taken orally as a drop or in water. It is very important to ONLY use the essential oils neat (no dilution) for those that are so indicated. Others will need to be diluted for either topical or oral use. Please also see Chapter 8 for a concise list of 12 essential oil remedies to consider for your essential oil travel first aid kit. The recommended amount of essential oil remedies should be listed on the package or container purchased, or commonly is only a drop or few drops at a time, whether used topically or internally.

Table 8.4 Essential oil first aid kit, 12 remedies : indications

Clove (*Syzygium aromaticum*) : Anti-inflammatory, antiseptic, anti-viral, anti-bacterial, anti-fungal anti-infectious, anti-parasitic, anti-aging, anti-oxidant, analgesic, anti-coagulant, immune stimulant, anticonvulsant, disinfectant, stomach protectant, warming.

Eucalyptus (*Eucalyptus globulus*) : Anti-viral, anti bacterial, anti-fungal, anti-aging, anti-infectious, anti-inflammatory, anti-rheumatic, antiseptic, deodorant, insecticidal, mucolytic, expectorant.

Frankincense (*Boswellia carterii*) : Anti-catarrhal, anti depressant, anti-infectious, antiseptic, expectorant, immune stimulant, muscle relaxant, sedative.

Helichrysum (*Helichrysum italicum*) : Anti-viral, anti inflammatory anti-spasmodic, expectorant, mucolytic, anesthetic, anti-coagulant, anti-catarrhal, anti-oxidant, liver stimulant/detoxifier, skin and nerve regenerator.

Lavender (*Lavandula angustifolia)* : Anti-fungal, analgesic, antiseptic, anti-convulsant, vasodilating, anti-spasmodic, anti-inflammatory, vermifuge.

Orange (*Citrus sinensis*) : Anti-septic, anti-depressant, anti spasmodic, digestive, circulatory stimulant, sedative, tonic.

Patchouli (*Pogostemon cablin*) : Anti-inflammatory, anti-fungal, anti-microbial,antiseptic, anti-toxic, astringent, decongestant, deodorant, diuretic, insecticidal, stimulant, relaxant, digestive aid, tonic.

Peppermint (*Mentha piperita*) : Anti-inflammatory, anti-viral, anti-parasitic, anti-bacterial, gallbladder, digestive stimulant, pain reliever, analgesic, anti-spasmodic.

Rosemary (*Rosmarinus officinalis*) : Anti-fungal, anti-bacterial, anti-viral, anti-parasitic, liver-protecting, cardio-tonic, digestive, detoxicant, anxiolytic.

Tea Tree *(Melaleuca alternifolia)* : Anti-viral, anti-bacterial, anti-fungal, anti-parasitic, antiseptic, anti-inflammatory, anti-oxidant, decongestant, immune-stimulant, insecticidal, tissue regenerator.

Ylang Ylang (*Cananga odorata*) : Anti-inflammatory, anti-spasmodic, antiseptic, anti- depressant, vasodilating, regulates heartbeat, anti-diabetic, tonic, sedative.

Blended essential oils:

Thieves® blend : Cinnamon Bark (*Cinnamonum verum)* : Antiseptic, anti-viral, anti-bacterial, anti-fungal, COX inhibitor (anti-inflammatory), strong oxygenator.

Clove (*Syzygium aromaticum*) : Antiseptic, anti-viral, anti-fungal, COX inhibitor

Eucalyptus (*Eucalyptus radiata)* : Anti-inflammatory, antiseptic, anti-viral, anti-bacterial, anti-fungal properties, supports respiratory system.

Lemon (*Citrus limon*) : Antiseptic, immune stimulating, purifying,uplifting.

Rosemary (*Rosmarius officinalis*) : Antiseptic, reduces mental fatigue, eases anxiety.

References

1. Alimi D, Geissmann A, Gardeur D. Acupuncture stimulation measured on functional magnetic resonance imaging. Medical Acupuncture 2002; 13: 18–21.
2. Arora DS, Kaur J. Antimicrobial activity of spices. International Journal of Antimicrobial Agents, 12 (1999): 257–262.
3. Auerbach PS (Ed). Wilderness Medicine, 6th Edition. Philadelphia, Mosby Elsevier, 2012.
4. Burnham T, et al (Eds). Drug Facts and Comparisons, St. Louis, Facts and Comparisons, 1999.
5. Dinsley J. CharcoalRemedies.com. The Complete Handbook of Medicinal Charcoal and its Applications. Coldwater, MI, Remnant Publications, 2005.
6. Duke JA. The Green Pharmacy: new discoveries in herbal remedies for common diseases and conditions from the nation's foremost authority on healing herbs. Emmaus, PA, Rodale Press, 1997.
7. Eisenberg DM, Davis RB, Ettner SL et al. Trends in alternative medicine use in the United States, 1990-1997: results of a follow-up national survey, JAMA 11 Nov 1998; 280(18): 1569-74.
8. Fenner PJ, Williamson JA, Burnett JW et al. First aid treatment of jellyfish stings in Australia: response to a newly differentiated species, Med J Aust 1993; 158:498.
9. Frank BL. 3-Phase Hand Therapy Reflex Chart. Edmond, OK, Acupuncture Medical Arts LLC, 2006.
10. Frank BL. An Integrated Approach to Pain and Sports Medicine. Thrive Oklahoma: Nurturing

References, continued

Body and Mind. Green Apple Publishing LLC 2011;2(5):37-38, 43.

11. Frank BL. Auricular Medicine and Auricular Therapy: A Practical Approach. Bloomington, IN, AuthorHouse, 2007.

12. Frank BL. Clinical case presentation: sports injury-alpine skiing. Medical Acupuncture. 1994;6(1):39.

13. Frank BL. Lighting the fire through acupuncture energetics: Jing Luo and beyond. Medical Acupuncture. 2005;17(1):13-17.

14. Frank BL. Medical acupuncture: a model of integrated healthcare from alternative to mainstream medicine. Colorado Medicine 1997; 94(7): 252-254.

15. Frank BL. Medical acupuncture and wilderness medicine: an integrated medical model in third world settings. Medical Acupuncture 1996; 8(1):11-15.

16. Frank BL. Medical acupuncture enhances standard wilderness care: a case study from the Inca Trail, Machu Picchu, Peru. Wilderness & Environmental Medicine 1998; 8(3): 161-163.

17. Frank BL. Neural Therapy. In Physical Medicine & Rehabilitation Clinics of North America. 1999;10(3):573-582.

18. Frank BL. Principles of Pain Management. In Wilderness Medicine, 5th Edition. Auerbach PS (Ed). St. Louis, Mosby, Inc., 2007.

19. Frank BL. The Layman's Guide to Auricular Therapy. Edmond, OK, Acupuncture Medical Arts, LLC, 2007.

20. Frank B. Silver as a Preferred Tool in International Medical Missions and Travel Medicine. In The

References, continued

Most Precious Metal : Why silver is more valuable than gold, platinum or money. Pedersen G. Pleasant Grove, UT, Silver Health Institute, 2013.

21. Frank BL, Soliman NE. Auricular Therapy Desk Reference Card. Edmond, OK, Acupuncture Arts & Press LLC, 2004.

22. Frank BL, Soliman NE. Hand Reflex Therapy Chart. Richardson, TX, Integrated Medicine Seminars LLC, 2002.

23. Frank BL, Soliman NE. Obesity treatment through auricular therapy and auricular medicine. Medical Acupuncture 2002;14(1):33-35.

24. Frank BL, Soliman NE. Shen Men: a critical assessment through advanced auricular therapy. Medical Acupuncture 1999; 10(2):17-19.

25. Frank BL, Soliman NE. Zero Point: a critical assessment through advanced auricular therapy. Medical Acupuncture 1999; 11(1):13-15.

26. Head H. On the disturbances of sensation, with special reference to the pain of visceral disease. Brain 1893; 16:1-133, Brain, 1894; 17:339-480, Brain 1896; 19:153-276.

27. Kenner D, Requena Y: Botanical Medicine: A European Professional Perspective, Brookline, MA, Paradigm Publications, 1996.

28. Kuusisto P, et al. Effect of activated charcoal on hypercholesterolemia. The Lancet, 16:366-7, August 1986.

29. Lednev LL. Possible mechanisms for the influence of weak magnetic fields on biological systems. Bioelectromagnetics 1991; 12:71-75.

Madigan SR, Raj PP. History and Current Status of Pain Management. In Raj PP (Ed): Practical of Pain,

References, continued

2nd edition, St. Louis, 1992, Mosby-Year Book, Inc.,1992.

30. McLean MJ et al. Blockage of sensory neuron action potentials by a static magnetic field in the 10mT range. Bioelectromagnetics 1995; 16:20-32.
31. Olney RK, So YT, Goodin DS, Aminoff MJ. A comparison of magnetic and electrical stimulation of peripheral nerves. Muscle & Nerve 1998; 11:21-32.
32. Nogier PFM. From Auriculotherapy to Auricular Medicine. Sainte-Ruffine, FR, Maisonneuve, 1983.
33. Nogier PFM. Handbook to Auriculotherapy. Sainte-Ruffine, FR, Maisonneuve, 1969.
34. Nogier PFM, Nogier R. The Man in the Ear. Sainte-Ruffine, FR, Maisonneuve, 1985.
35. Pedersen G. A New Fighting Chance: Silver Solution, 4th Edition. Pleasant Grove, UT, GP Silver LLC, 2014.
36. Pedersen G. The Most Precious Metal : Why Silver is More Valuable Than Gold, Platinum or Money. Pleasant Grove, UT, Silver Health Institute, 2013.
37. Pedersen. The Silver Solution to Women's Wellness : using the new Structured Silver for all areas of female health, 2nd Edition. Pleasant Grove, UT, Silver Health Institute, 2013.
38. Pedersen G, Hegde BM. Silver sol completely removes malaria parasites from the blood of human subjects infected with malaria in an average of five days : A review of four randomized, multi-centered, clinical studies performed in Africa. The Indian Practitioner 2010 ;63 (9) :567-574.
39. Price P, Price S. Aromatherapy for Babies and Children. Stratford-upon-Avon, England, Riverhead Publishing, 2005.

References, continued

40. Saberski LR. Cryoneurolysis in Clinical Practice. In Waldman SD, Winnie AP: Interventional Pain Management, Philadelphia, WB Saunders Co., 1996.
41. Smith PW. What You Must Know About Vitamins, Minerals, Herbs & More. New Hyde Park, NY, Square One Publishers, 2008.
42. Smith PW. What You Must Know About Women's Hormones: Your Guide to Natural Hormone Treatments for PMS, Menopause, Osteoporosis, PCOS and More. New Hyde Park, NY, Square One Publishers, 2009.
43. Soliman NE, Frank BL. Soliman-Frank 3-Phase hand acupuncture. Medical Acupuncture 2005;17(1):29-34.
44. Soliman NE, Frank BL. Auricular Acupuncture and Auricular Medicine. In Physical Medicine & Rehabilitation Clinics of North America.1999;10(2) :547-554.
45. Stengler M. The Nataural Physician's Healing Therapies. Paramus, NJ, Prentice Hall, 2001.
46. Vasudevan S, et al. Physical Methods of Pain Management. In Raj PP (ed): Practical Management of Pain, 2nd edition, St. Louis, Mosby-Year Book, Inc., 1992.
47. Weintraub MI. Chronic submaximal magnetic stimulation in peripheral neuropathy: is there a beneficial therapeutic relationship? AJPM 1998; 8(1):12-16.

Text Figures, Tables and Titles

Text Figures, Tables and Titles, continued

Frank BL: Medical acupuncture and wilderness medicine: an integrated medical model in third world settings. Medical Acupuncture 1996; 8(1):11-15.

Figure 7.2 Hand Therapy reflex charts
Frank BL, Soliman NE. Hand Reflex Therapy Chart. Richardson, TX, Integrated Medicine Seminars LLC, 2002.

Figure 7.3 Hand Therapy advanced phases charts
Frank BL. 3-Phase Hand Therapy Reflex Chart. Edmond, OK, Acupuncture Medical Arts LLC, 2006.

Figure 7.4 "Inverted Fetus"
Frank BL. Auricular Medicine and Auricular Therapy: A Practical Approach. Bloomington, IN, AuthorHouse, 2007.

Figure 7.5 Phase 1 auricular projections
Frank BL, Soliman NE. Auricular Therapy Desk Reference Card. Edmond, OK, Acupuncture Arts & Press LLC, 2004.

Table 8.1 Essential First Aid Kit. ALWAYS carry
Table 8.2 Botanical/herbal First Aid kit, 12 remedies : indications
Table 8.3 Homeopathic First Aid kit, 12 remedies : indications
Table 8.4 Essential oil First Aid kit, 12 remedies : indications

Resources for Information or Products

Acupuncture Medical Arts, LLC (also called:
Acupuncture Arts & Press LLC and Integrated Medicine
Seminars LLC)
P.O. Box 851952
Yukon, OK 73085-1952 USA
www.AuricularTherapy.com
Acupuncture, auricular therapy, hand therapy texts, atlases,
charts, supplies, and seminars.

BioThera International, LLC
P.O. Box 851952
Yukon, OK 73085-1952
www.stonemillventures.com
Structured Silver for lay and professionals and other natural
health products.

American Academy of Anti-Aging & Regenerative
Medicine (A4M)
1801 N. Military Trail, Suite 200
Boca Raton, FL 33431
www.a4m.com
Integrative training, education and Board Certification for
healthcare professionals.

American Academy of Medical Acupuncture (AAMA)
4929 Wilshire Boulevard, #428
Los Angeles, CA 90010 USA
www.medicalacupuncture.org
Membership organization for medical acupuncturists,
seminars and symposia, professional journal.

Resources for Information or Products, continued

American Association of Acupuncture and Oriental
Medicine (AAAOM)
P.O. Box 162340
Sacramento, CA 95816 USA
www.aaom.org
Membership association for licensed and registered
acupuncturists, seminars and congresses.

American Medical College of Homeopathy
2001 W. Camelback Road, Suite 150
Phoenix, AZ 85015
www.AMCofH.org
Professional training in classical homeopathy.

Apex Energetics
16592 Hale Ave.
Irvine, CA 92606
www.apexenergetics.com
Quality homeopathic remedies for professionals, seminars,
information.

BoironUSA
6 Campus Boulevard
Newtown Square, PA 19073-3267
www.boironusa.com
World leader in homeopathic remedies.

BuyActivatedCharcoal.com
P.O. Box 261
Crawford, NE 69339
www.BuyActivatedCharcoal.com
Quality activated charcoal products and information.

Resources for Information or Products, continued

Experience Essential Oils
www.experience-essential-oils.com
Extensive web resource and single and blended essential oils.

Haus Bioceuticals
755 Research Parkway
Oklahoma City, OK 73104-1232
www.hausbio.com/TravelDoc
Evidence-based biological remedies for eczema, psoriasis, diabetic ulcers, bedsores, ultra-soluble curcumin and more.

Heel, Inc.
10421 Research Road SE
Albuquerque, NM 87123-3423
www.heelusa.com
Advanced homeopathic remedies, including Traumeel® and Zeel®.

Helio Medical Supplies
606 Charcot Avenue
San Jose, CA 95131 USA
www.heliomed.com
Comprehensive acupuncture supplies and resources.

Homeodynamics, LLC
P.O. Box 44275
Madison, WI 53744-4275
www.homeodynamics.com
Advanced homeopathic and homeodynamic remedies for professional providers.

Resources for Information or Products, continued

Kan Herb Company
380 Encinal Street, Suite 100
Santa Cruz, CA 95060
www.kanherb.com
Herbal remedies for consumers and professionals.

Katadyn Products Inc.
Pfäffikerstrasse 37
8310 Kemptthal
Switzerland
www.katadyngroup.com
Premier water filtration equipment.

Lhasa OMS Medical Supplies, Inc.
230 Libbey Parkway
Weymouth, MA 02189 USA
www.lhasaoms.com
Comprehensive acupuncture supplies and resources.

MVT PRA
Micro-Vibrational Therapy - Personal Relief Assistant
2110 Pinto Lane
Las Vegas, NV
www.mvtpra.com
Natural micro-vibrational pain relief therapy units.

Nelsons Natural World
21 High Street, Suite 302
North Andover, MA 01845
www.nelsonsnaturalworld.com
150+-year supplier of homeopathic, Bach Flower remedies.

Resources for Information or Products, continued

REI
Sumner, WA 98352-0001
www.rei.com
Classic outdoor activity supplier, water filter supplies, etc.

Silver Health Institute
898 South Main
Pleasant Grove, UT 84062
www.silverhealthinstitute.com
Advanced silver products information, webinars, video teaching, books.

Silver Resonance, Inc.
ThankYouSilver.com, Structured Silver for consumers. Please use DISCOUNT CODE 54321 for orders online. pHStructuredSilver.com, Structured Silver for professionals, extensive resources. USE REFERRAL CODE BIOTHERA

Structured Silver for Consumers:
www.TravelDoc.info

Structured Silver for Professionals:
www.TravelDoc.info

Wilderness Medical Society
2150 S 1300 E, Suite 500
Salt Lake City, Utah 84106
www.wms.org
Leader in medical/allied medical wilderness medicine training and education, publications.

Resources for Information or Products, continued

Young Living, Inc.
Thanksgiving Point Business Park
3125 Executive Parkway
Lehi, UT 84043
www.youngliving.com
Extensive web information, single or blended essential oils.
Please use Sponsor Code: 1929743 when you enroll.

Zeo Health Ltd.
159 Route 303
Valley Cottage, NY 10989
Original Zeolite products and information.

Made in the USA
San Bernardino, CA
13 August 2014